A CRITICAL A-Z (

Craig Newnes has many selves including author, editor, musician, independent scholar, dad, gardener and Consulting Critical Psychologist. Until retiring after a near-fatal road accident, he was a Consultant Clinical Psychologist and Director of Psychological Therapies for Shropshire's Mental Health (NHS) Trust and Chair of the British Psychological Society Psychotherapy Section. He has published numerous book chapters and academic articles and is editor of *The Journal of Critical Psychology, Counselling and Psychotherapy*. His books include *Clinical Psychology: A critical examination* and the edited volumes: *Children in Society: Politics, policies and interventions, Making and Breaking Children's Lives; Spirituality and Psychotherapy; This is Madness: A critical look at psychiatry and the future of mental health services; This is Madness Too: A further critical look at mental health services* all from PCCS Books. His latest books are *Inscription, Diagnosis and Deception in the Mental Health Industry: How Psy governs us all* (Palgrave Macmillan: 2016) and an edited collection, *Teaching Critical Psychology: International perspectives* (Routledge: 2018). With his dad he has written a book on the Malaysian Emergency; *Malaya*. His novels *Paris* and *Tearagh't* are published by The Real Press and tracks from his band *Sandghosts* are available from Amazon.

.

A Critical A-Z
of Electroshock

Craig Newnes

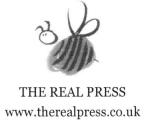

THE REAL PRESS
www.therealpress.co.uk

Published in 2018 by the Real Press.
www.therealpress.co.uk
© Craig Newnes

ISBN (print) 9781912119523
ISBN (ebooks) 9781912119738

To May – long may you run!

Acknowledgements

Thank you to survivors, activists, friends, colleagues and authors Viv Lindow, Olive Bucknall, Lucy Johnstone, Peter Lehmann, Peter Breggin, the late Judi Chamberlain, Steve Baldwin, Mark Rapley and Leonard Roy Frank, to Joe Grace for research on 'Fits and Frances Farmer' and 'Queerness', to David Boyle for keeping the faith, to Isabel and my long-suffering family and to all those in cyberspace and elsewhere who do their best.

Contents

Foreword

My earliest encounter with electroshock (at the time called Electroconvulsive Therapy) was as a clinical psychology student, filled with curiosity and too naïve to question my instructions to be an observer.

As I recall, it wasn't like I'd seen in the films – particularly as the relatively junior psychiatrist embarking on the second step of the 'see one, do one, teach one' learning cycle, managed to first shock himself before the patient. Aside from this introduction more dramatic even than any film could provide, what stood out for me was the assuredness of the staff at every stage of the process. Also, their confidence that shock was going to be 'helpful' for the patient (whatever helpful meant); and their certainty that any disorientation, confusion and memory loss was guaranteed to be temporary.

This was a sharp needle to my bubble of naivety. How can one ever be so certain and hold such faith in anything? I came to know Craig Newnes years later as a member of the editorial collective for *Clinical Psychology Forum,* for which he was the co-ordinating editor for almost 20 years. Craig was and has remained a significant influence on my thinking; encouraging my desire to question and explore the hidden depths and complexities that lie beyond the face value of what is before us.

Many assume that to be critical is to be biased in

perspective, closed down, reductionist and misleading. Yet, to be truly critical, it requires one to really look at something with sustained attention and an openness that permits observation from every available angle. It requires a genuine curiosity that brings with it an in-depth understanding and generates broader perspectives.

This is exactly what I love about the way Craig thinks about something, which he expresses so eloquently as a writer – his ability to take you on a journey that starts with lifting the lid of a Pandora's box and then navigating you through an eclectic mix of discoveries that are unravelled and deconstructed before your eyes.

It's a kind of experiential storytelling where, as you are tempted into indulging in an array of fascinations and curiosities, you suddenly find yourself challenged by questioning what you weren't aware of wanting to question.

This *A-Z of Electroshock* is a magnificent example of such a journey. It is wonderful collection of history, fact and trivia expertly weaved into an informed, positioned perspective on the world of Psy. For any student this will provide a valuable introduction that will form bridges to a wealth of knowledge acquired through years of experience.

For anyone who considers themselves more knowledgeable or expert in the field, this will be a polemical deconstruction of electroshock that redirects your awareness to new perspectives and insights. The praxis has always been a source of debate and controversy To quote Albert Einstein, we can't solve problems by using the same kind of thinking we used when we created them, and in this A-Z, Craig Newnes provides a very new kind of thinking.

Dr Sara Tai, Consultant Clinical Psychologist and Senior Lecturer in Clinical Psychology, University of Manchester.

Introduction

To the surprise of many, electroshock (promoted as Electro-convulsive *Therapy*) remains a core intervention in psychiatry, especially for older women. Its reputation as alternatively 'life-saving' and 'barbaric' ensures that the public remains largely ignorant of its potential for harm and television documentaries tend to be neutral on the topic.

It is a practice hidden behind the closed doors of the clinic, one well known to in-patient psychiatric staff (though ignored by most community psy professionals) and rarely publicised despite at least one psychiatric journal being entirely devoted to the practice. The occasional television documentary, radio interview or TED Talk rehashes variants on 'progress' versus the horrors of *One Flew Over the Cuckoo's Nest*.

The ancient Egyptians used electric marine rays to treat epilepsy and the ancient Romans used the current generated by electric eels for the treatment of headaches, gout, and to assist in obstetric procedures. The journal *Electricity and Medicine* was first published in 1744. It was claimed that electric stimuli could be curative for 'neurologic and mental cases of paralysis and epilepsy'.[1]

In the 1755 edition, J. B. LeRoy detailed a case of hysterical blindness cured with three applications of electric shock and in 1752 Benjamin Franklin had recorded the use of an 'electro static machine to cure a woman of hysterical fits'.[2] By the mid-nineteenth century Duchenne, the 'father of electrotherapy', was to say, 'No sincere neurologist could practice without the use of electrotherapy.'[3]

There lies the rub. Duchenne was a neurologist, a branch of medicine specializing in real, frequently directly observable, assaults to the brain – carcinoma, head injury, stroke and so on. Psychiatry and psychology, however, deal exclusively in metaphor and a never-ending attempt to classify conduct and delineate certain behaviours or characteristics as 'mad' or 'symptoms of mental illness.' There is no neurological basis for psychiatric categories, nor could there ever be. Psychiatry and psychology operate in the world of linguistics and metaphor – neurologists and the rest of us operate in the real world.

If you are an inscribed (diagnosed) person looking for solace in what follows, you may be disappointed as the magic of diagnosis and so-called treatment are stripped bare. If you are a psy professional committed to doing your best on behalf of your patients, you should give them a copy. If you believe electrocution can benefit an organ as complex and sensitive as the brain this volume will expose the myths surrounding its use.

Those myths include different accounts of its invention, the idea it is a life-saver, the notion that shock induced convulsions are more important than the shock itself, claims concerning its safety, lack of adverse effects, and absence of vested interest in its prescription and the false claim that it is primarily given to those described as depressed as a 'treatment of last resort.' Myths and self-deception are useful ways to keep our heads above water in an uncertain world. *A Critical A-Z of Electroshock* may not be comfortable reading – but it may prevent you drowning in illusion.

Totalitarianism cannot tolerate jokes – self-depreciating humour is *verboten*. It relies on lies rather than laughter. Mao, Stalin, Hitler and Elizabeth I were not noted for their humour; though Judi Dench's portrayal of Queen Bess in *Shakespeare in Love* has its moments. She also once described the bard as 'the man who pays the rent.'[4]

Governments, systems of governmentality and professions are similarly po-faced. There are few laugh-out-loud moments in a volume such as this but it is worth remembering that the pursuit of 'cure' for non-existent illness described at all times as conditions (effectively, just the way people live their lives) is farcical. Have I told you the one about...? Psy-recipients and activists can likewise be accused of a certain sanctimony though there are exceptions; Woody Allen has made a career out of his experience of analysis. Freud was compelled to see humour as a much darker instrument.

Perhaps, 'what I am doing is entertainment. Choose between an entertaining life and the other kind - or the 'art' life. The answer becomes obvious.'[5] Readers might like to approach this A-Z in random order. Or, start with the letters that spell out your first name. For the author that would imply C (Consent and Clementine Churchill), R (Research and Robeson), A (Assault and

Antonin Artaud), I (Inscription and Insulin coma) and G (Governmentality and Gene Tierney). Or, perhaps, 'Start at the very beginning. It's a very good place to start.'[6]

Assault and Antonin Artaud

Assault in health services frequently hits the headlines. This is usually criminal assault, often involving violence against, or by, patients and staff. This first entry in this volume, however, is about assaults on people and ensuing harm that is a normal part of psychiatric treatment.

Jung suggested that we only learn through our mistakes: watch a seven-year-old try to nip out a candle flame without wetting her fingers and then watch her do it a second time having first licked her finger-tips. Falling off bicycles, stepping on hot sand and touching a bare electric live wire come into the same category. Sadly, we frequently don't learn through our errors; starting a new relationship with an aggressive partner having recently finished a relationship with an aggressive person is but one of many examples. As a species we seem doomed to repeat mistakes and rarely learn from the mistakes made by others.

The child psychotherapist Donald Winnicott claimed that destructiveness was an integral part of creation – an artist, for example, destroys a blank canvas whilst simultaneously creating a painting.

Making errors from which we may not learn and the destructiveness inherent to creativity are cardinal features of medical procedures. A surgeon must first anaesthetise a patient (with all the inherent risks of anaesthesia) before cutting through healthy tissue in order to perform what may be a life-saving operation, a general practitioner may prescribe several different drugs or dosages before arriving at a prescription involving less adverse effects.

The kind of experimentation common to medicine can be regarded as a form of assault though the intention is benign and the outcome frequently to the patient's benefit. For people with the power to consent such assault is mitigated by giving as much information as possible (see Consent and Clementine Churchill).

As a branch of medicine psychiatry finds itself with historic, epistemological and scientific reasons for a rigorous self-examination of whether its procedures should be regarded as non-benign assault rather than helpful treatment. For many a combination of repeated mistakes and destructiveness pushes the discipline into the former rather than latter category.

As Thomas Szasz puts it:

'The reality of psychiatric coercion and dehumanization is camouflaged by...a lexicon of euphemisms concealing the exploitation and injury of so called mental patients as 'treatments'.[1]

Two-and-a-half thousand years ago, Sushruta, a Hindu physician, claimed that madness was caused by 'strong emotions and passions'.[2] Plato, over a hundred years later, suggested madness occurred when the rational soul (located in the brain) was separated from the irrational soul (located in the chest, close to the heart). By 100 BCE, Soranus was using these ideas to recommend service rather than control, and the use of a tranquil ground-floor lighted room.[3] He argued against restraint and recommended talking to patients about what interested them.

From antiquity, physicians intent on changing mood recommended a mixture of more gentle praxis (especially for the rich) and more potentially destructive treatments. Soranus, in addition to a light diet, exercise and music, suggested blood-letting, leeches and poultices to counteract the black bile of melancholia. The regime was derived from Celsus, a follower of Hippocrates.[4]

So many people were deemed mad and incarcerated during the nineteenth century that the development of means to control unruly inmates became of great concern to asylum superintendents and medical staff. For nursing staff, assault by patients due to overcrowded conditions was a daily risk. Except for the more resistant patients, straitjackets were rapidly superseded by drugs including bromides, cocaine, caffeine, paraldehyde and the sulphonamides.

By the mid-twentieth century, psychiatric inmates were being assaulted with metrazol, insulin, psychosurgery, major tranquillizers such as lithium and chlorpromazine (marketed as drugs to combat supposed conditions such as manic depression and schizophrenia), and electroshock (called Electroconvulsive *Therapy* and marketed as a specific treatment for schizophrenia and depression for an age range of 4–104).[5]

Today the promotion of ideas like 'mental ill-health' and 'well-being' leads increasing numbers to seek counselling, meditation and medication to ease what Freud called ordinary human misery. An electrified form of psychosurgery is still practised and electroshock continues to be marketed for those inscribed with autism, depression, schizophrenia and other psychiatric terms depending on where you happen to live and your power to resist.

Antonin Artaud

The playwright and founder of the absurdist Theatre of Cruelty, Antonin Artaud was prescribed Laudanum at a sanatorium in 1919. He became a lifelong heroin addict. After returning from Ireland in 1937, Artaud spent the last years of his life in different French asylums inscribed with schizophrenia and 'graphorrhea'.

In 1943, friends of Artaud had him transferred to the psychiatric hospital in Rodez under Dr Gaston Ferdière who prescribed 58 electroshock bursts. Ferdière had come to Paris as a young idealistic poet and, as an intern at Sainte Anne, had worked with 'Professor Claude,' whom Breton pilloried in the anti-psychiatric Nadja. In Paris, he met Desnos, Péret, Michaux, and René Crevel, who confessed his despair to the young psychiatrist over drinks on the eve of his suicide.

Food supplies had been severely curtailed by the Nazis in the Occupied territories, and thousands of mental patients starved. An outspoken critic of this policy, Ferdière worked the black market to supply inmates with food at Rodez, and Artaud recovered from the brink of starvation.

Ferdière's interest in poetry was rekindled in conversations with Artaud, whose literary talents he sought to restore through 'art therapy' (writing, drawing and translating *Through the Looking Glass*) accompanied by electroshock between June 20, 1943 and January 24, 1945. The intensity of Artaud's delusions increased, as did the quality of the 'magical' drawings and incantations he drew.

Ferdière believed that Artaud's habits of crafting magic spells, creating astrology charts, and drawing disturbing images were symptoms of mental illness. In 1946, Ferdière released Artaud to his friends who placed him in the psychiatric clinic at Ivry-sur-Seine. He died shortly afterwards on 4 March 1948, alone. It was suspected that he died from a lethal dose of chloral hydrate, although it is unknown whether he was aware of its lethality.

Soon after the electroshock he had written: 'Anyone who has gone through the electric shock ... never again rises out of its darkness and his life has been lowered a notch.'[6]

Bystanders and Bud Powell

Electroshock might be viewed as representative of much that occurs within the Psy complex: the technique has harmed millions; it is based on suspect and ever-changing theoretical assumptions; research is scientistic and carried out frequently by those with vested interests in the results; it is most commonly used on those with little power who have been marked, frequently via psychometric assessment, in the context of coercion and lack of consent; and – importantly – health professionals are largely silent on the topic. For Erwin Staub, they would be classed as 'bystanders' in the face of harm perpetrated on patients in the same system within which they work.[1]

Many service recipient groups and activists speak out about electroshock; on Facebook pages, via net-based support groups, in conferences and in print (see Opposition and Oprah Winfrey). Psychiatrists such as Peter Breggin have argued passionately and authoritatively against electroshock since the 1970s.[2] Some clinical psychologists have been equally outspoken.[3]

For the majority of mental health professionals, however, electroshock remains invisible and, like the general public, new entrants to the psy professions are surprised to find it still exists. Although ignorance is no defence – especially in post-doctoral disciplines where informed critique should be the norm – those that don't know about electroshock are not, technically, bystanders.

There remain, however, thousands of psy workers – from social work staff to clinical psychologists – who know about the practice and do nothing. In Goldie's term these workers are in the 'compliant' position.[4] It is a position that serves psy professionals well. The desire to get on with fellow professionals in closed social groups (ward rounds, case conferences, etc.) dulls any protest. Professional self-interest makes complicity and active participation in electroshock highly likely. For example, nurses training in psychiatry must witness it before actively participating in its delivery.

In similar vein, clinical psychologists use psychometrics and interviews to arrive at a diagnosis (see Inscription and Insulin coma) supporting psychiatric nosology and praxis. If a person is inscribed as depressed by a psycho-diagnostic procedure then, depending on their sex, age, the preferences of the consultant psychiatrist (see Zealotry and Zelda Fitzgerald) and other factors they may be electroshocked.

Psychology and clinical psychology in particular are held within something of a trap as by-standing disciplines due, in part, to their claims to be sciences. Though the scientific project is bounded by economic and disciplinary imperatives it is frequently claimed to be morally neutral. Scientists tend not to examine the distal forces dictating what can be studied and, for psychology, the need to be seen as a science has tended to prevent many psychologists questioning their role as allies of medicine.

The position is summarised in the editorial of the first edition of the *British Journal of Psychology*:

> 'Psychology ... known among us as mental philosophy ... has now achieved the position of a positive science ... 'Ideas' in the philosophical sense do not fall within its scope; its enquiries are restricted entirely to facts.'[5]

It is, perhaps, ironic that one renowned psychologist writes: 'Psychology has yet to establish a single fact about human behaviour.'[6] As a science, psychology has failed; but as an unchallenged discourse it reigns supreme. Weber had a pessimistic view of science itself: 'Science is meaningless because it gives no answers to our question, the only question important for us: 'What shall we do and how shall we live?' '[7]

The allegiance to medicine is made explicit by the statement of purpose of the *Journal of Clinical Psychology*. Since 1945, readers have been informed that the journal is, 'a monthly peer reviewed *medical* journal covering psychological research, assessment, and practice...It covers research on psychopathology, psychodiagnostics, psychotherapy, psychological assessment and treatment matching, clinical outcomes, clinical health psychology, and behavioural medicine' (my emphasis).

In such a professional context, bystanding becomes

the norm. In a work context standing by may feel like the only option for a professional without allies. For example, a job description attached to a recent advertisement for a medical 'Foundation Placement' in the Merseycare NHS Trust (based in Liverpool, UK) states: 'Opportunities exist for training by the Clinical Psychologist, observe ECT, have taster sessions at a community clinic, etc.' It is telling that the training opportunity from the clinical psychologist is placed adjacent to electroshock observation.

In the context of training or a psy professional's early career, compliance is often through active engagement, participation that the professional may come to regret. Szasz quotes R.D. Laing: 'As a young psychiatrist ... I administered locked wards and ordered drugs, padded cells and straitjackets, electric shock, deep insulin comas, and the rest.'[9]

Peter Breggin, one of the foremost psychiatrists critical of electroshock said:

'As I look back on my career as a psychiatrist, one shame seems unforgivable – my involvement with electroshock treatment. As a resident in psychiatry, I prescribed electroshock, I supervised a ward on which patients were given the treatment, and for a time I personally administered it. Why, then, did I do it even if I knew it was wrong?'[10]

Laing and Breggin are not alone in collaborating with the administration of electroshock. As part of the training of psychiatrists participation has been inevitable for the majority. It is one aspect of psychiatry's continuing struggle to prove itself a branch of physical medicine through its use of physical interventions. But the existence of electroshock is not commented on by numerous leading psychiatric and psychological theorists and practitioners. Aaron Beck (the originator of Cognitive Behaviour Therapy - CBT) and Carl Rogers don't mention it, mirroring the silence from psy professionals around the world. Rogers, in particular, was pilloried by Jeffrey Masson in *Against Therapy* for condoning the plight of people inscribed with schizophrenia in the wards where he carried out his early research on person-centred counselling.

Like Rogers, many counsellors and psychotherapists are too busy pursuing cultural capital to speak out. Electroshock isn't in the index of the monumental *History of Psychotherapy*.[11]

More typically, psychiatric historian Michael Stone's equally thorough *Healing the Mind* mentions it only briefly as a successful treatment for depression and schizophrenia.[12] As ever in psy theorizing, theorists and practitioners are unwilling to use their own theories in a reflexive manner; psycho-analytic psychiatrists don't see prescribing electroshock as a form of sadism (see Sadism and Spike Milligan), other professionals don't see by-standing in terms of the difficulty of speaking out in groups (for example, ward rounds; though Lucy Johnstone is an exception[13]) and practitioners of cognitive behaviour therapy (CBT) don't examine the cognitive distortion within their belief that electroshock works - they fail to examine the evidence against their belief despite witnessing the deleterious effects of electrocution on their patients.

Clinical psychologist and doyenne of the self-help movement Dorothy Rowe (who was 87 the day I wrote this) established the UK's North Lincolnshire Department of Clinical Psychology in 1972. The Department had its offices (actually a portakabin) in the grounds of St John's Hospital, Bracebridge Heath near Lincoln.

In 1983, Dorothy won the MIND book of the year award with *Depression: The way out of your prison.* She usually comes across in person and print as certain but can be curiously ambivalent about electroshock:

> 'My depressed clients often ask me what I think of ECT and whether I would advise them to have it. My answer is that ordinarily I would not approve of a person having his chest cut open or being thumped heavily and persistently on the chest, but when these are ways to get the heart functioning again, then of course I approve. ECT has an equally dramatic and usually successful life-saving effect on a person who has become so depressed that he is immobile and starving or agitated to the point of exhaustion ... you cannot live your life hoping that every time you get depressed someone will give you ECT ... you have to alter your way of living...'[14]

This ambivalence is contextual. In part both Rowe and the patient are contextualized by their relationship – Dorothy is meant to give sensible advice that the patient can follow; the patient is not meant to say, 'Change my life! Are you serious? ECT is easier.' In part the ambivalence may be a product of Rowe's working environment. When built in 1852 as Lincolnshire Lunatic Asylum, St John's hospital held 250 patients. By 1926 the site had been expanded to cover 160 acres. Briefly, between the wars it was renamed Bracebridge Mental Hospital and at its height the building had 944 beds, four times the original size. Electroshock was a favoured intervention for the in-patients.

The Lincolnshire clinical psychologists were principally involved in developing primary care services to GPs, a position that made it difficult to challenge the hospital practice of electroshock; they were, in effect, bystanders.

The hospital closed in 1990 and by 2011 electroshock was being given at the Peter Hodgkinson Centre (under the auspices of the Lincolnshire Partnership NHS Foundation Trust) to around 80 people annually. A third of treatments were compulsory. An article in the local GP newsletter dealing with mental health and similar services claims a two thirds success rate for electro-shock and includes the – now common – feel-good story about a grateful, fully recovered female electroshock recipient from the author's earlier days as a registrar.[15]

Bud Powell

'If I had to choose one single musician for his artistic integrity, for the incomparable originality of his creation and the grandeur of his work, it would be Bud

Powell. He was in a class by himself.'[16]

Earl Rudolph 'Bud' Powell (September 27, 1924 – July 31, 1966) was an American jazz pianist, born and raised in Harlem, New York City. It is claimed that by the time of the Second World War he was rivalling his hero, Art Tatum. His contract with the Coolie Williams swing orchestra was terminated in January 1945, when he was apprehended, drunk, by the private railroad police. He was beaten and then briefly incarcerated. Ten days after his release he was hospitalized; first in Bellevue on an observation ward and then in a state psychiatric hospital sixty miles away. He stayed there for two and a half months.

He went on to record with, amongst others, Dexter Gordon, Charlie Parker, Sarah Vaughan and Miles Davis and in 1947 after another drunken fight he was sent to Bellevue and then Creedmore State Hospital (see Law and Lou Reed). He stayed for eleven months and frequently complained of racism.[17]

He was given electroshock from February to April and then a second, equally unsuccessful series in May. Further incarcerations interrupted his recording career. By the late 1950s, now taking the tranquillizing neuroleptic Chlorpromazine, although his composing continued his playing was seriously affected. Still taking Chlorpromazine Powell moved to Paris in 1959 with Altevia 'Buttercup' Edwards, a fellow patient from 1954.[18] He returned to New York in 1964 eventually being re-hospitalized. On July 31, 1966, he died of tuberculosis, malnutrition, and alcoholism; thousands came to his funeral procession in Harlem.

Consent and
Clementine Churchill

Schopenhauer said: 'Life is farce disguised as tragedy.' There are few professions with as much to gain as psy from the presentation of ordinary human misery as tragic and the farcical attempts to alleviate it as heroic.

Adding insult to injury are the extraordinary efforts of the psy survivor movement and its various professional allies to lock horns with the monolith that is the modern psy industry. Hundreds of thousands of people try to make this scientistic enterprise accountable and 'better' as if praxis with governmentality at its heart could be better. People become exhausted in an essentially farcical enterprise (see Opposition and Oprah Winfrey).

The way in which consent (or lack of it) and conflict of interest interact in this endeavour bears scrutiny. *Great and Desperate Cures* is one of the best titles to be found in the psy canon.[1] It simultaneously expresses the cultural capital to be found in the trope of 'greatness,' the two-sided meaning of the word desperate (terrified and ridiculous) and the idea that psy involves 'cure.'

But cure for what? Is there a cure for unhappiness, for refusing to eat, for disturbing others through one's conduct or declarations? These are all socially embedded experiences. Happiness is constantly in flux – from moment to moment we can be happy, sad, indifferent, and, depending on our circumstances, some feelings will predominate for longer than others. Refusing to eat isn't a crime. It can be a protest (as in the case of the Maze prison hunger-strikers in County Down; Bobby Sands died in May 1981 after refusing to eat for 66 days), an extreme form of dieting and something a child does to show a parent how cross he or she is. It is, however, frequently distressing – read infuriating, alarming, and guilt-provoking – to those around the self-starver. Scratching, cutting wrists, hair-pulling, and throwing fits of melancholy or rage are pretty disturbing too. Adults not involved in warfare or terrorism shouting out that G-d has told them to kill or take their clothes off in a shopping mall can be terrifying.

Changing this kind of intentional behaviour is fraught with complications. If the conduct is inscribed as a disorder or condition, the responsibility for invoking change is removed to a professional. Professionals could describe themselves as 'individual or system change agents.' This would imply that they can actually change intentional conduct. Instead, they elect themselves 'therapists' or enter a professional scheme of governmentality such as psychiatry or one of the several sub-disciplines of psychology. At this point 'change' becomes 'personal development', 'growth', 'recovery' or 'cure'.

Valenstein's title neatly summarises over a century of peoples' efforts to change the lives of others; and these lives - sad or mad though they may appear - are simply the way people live. Psy attempts to cure us of life – a desperate ambition indeed. It is an ambition mirrored in the work of politicians, faith-healers, priests, advertising executives and the interrelated schemes and actions inherent to social existence. Road-builders and town and country planners have the power to change the lives of others through community friendly or unfriendly design. Armaments manufacturers have the power to benefit or destroy millions. Here lies the irony of psy's desperation.

Psy has singularly failed to make the lives of people much better and, in the case of the 'cures' outlined in this and similar volumes, has been a powerful force for harm. How could it be otherwise? People inscribed by psy are not 'ill.' They are troublesome and soon become unwanted (unless they change). Psy intervenes and for consenting adults the game commences: I pretend I want to change, but can't – You pretend you can change me, but can't. For minors and those subjected to psy against their will, the game is more honest: I don't want to change, and won't – You are paid to do this, good luck.

For the first two hundred years of institutional psychiatry (a period that pre-dated any 'profession' of psychology), concerns about consent were largely absent. Pauper lunatics were housed in asylums to prevent them disturbing the peace and many rich patients were sent to private institutions by relatives disturbed by their conduct. Then, as now, children and weak or dementing older persons were not in a position to give consent. For incarcerated adults, inscription was followed by 'treatments' indistinguishable from punishment. Some, like plunging patients into icy water required a lack of consent (or the surprise element would be lost). Others – isolation and mechanical or chemical restraint – were used to prevent patients causing too much disharmony in the hospitals. Again, consent was not a concern. For patients fortunate enough to come across a medical superintendent keen to try moral therapy or a talking cure, consent was implied.

Neither moral therapy nor kindly conversations had specific parameters so patients couldn't have known what they were consenting to. Again, this still obtains in contemporary versions of psychotherapy and counselling; relationships are unique so neither therapist nor patient can reliably predict what will happen.

The so called innovation or 'heroism' of doctors prepared to take risks with the lives of their patients is eloquently summarised by Medawar: '...professional attitudes towards the mentally ill ...reflect deep-seated notions of illness as an expression of personal fate and of medical treatment as the next best thing to divine intervention.'[2] The position obtains in all aspects of psy – from therapists who *charge* for talking to people to otherwise unemployable thirty-somethings who take *courses* to become 'healers.'

As a psychiatrist himself, Berne inverted the exploitative arrogance of psy professionals by naming the game from the patient's perspective: 'Gee you're wonderful professor.'[3] Nonetheless it would be a singularly modest professional who did not respond to a patient's adulation, especially if the perceived esteem was backed up by payment. In the case of electroshock, such dynamics have largely been irrelevant. Since its inception, it has been foisted on people in a wholly experimental manner. Many recipients have no power to object and many others might describe themselves as 'desperate.'

In the first years following Bini and Cerletti's design and production of an electroshock device, ten per cent of US institutions had replaced cardiazol shock with electroshock. The Bethlehem Royal Hospital took delivery of its first electroshock machine in 1940. Results were claimed to be 'very satisfactory.'[4] On visiting, with his own machine, St Ebba's Hospital Epsom William Sargant (who Fennell suggests saw medical heroism as overcoming bureaucracy to bring patients, '... the latest available treatment.'[5]) asked to see some 'agitated depressives.' He then gave almost an entire ward electroshocks. Informed consent was not considered – not least because Sargant didn't know what would happen.

'Consent' as such was not seen as an issue in the UK until the 1970s. Until that decade, doctors operated under a principle established in 1957 by the case of *Bolam v Friern Hospital Management Committee*. A patient undergoing unmodified electroshock claimed that the psychiatrist had broken his duty of care when he failed to disclose the risks common to not using a muscle relaxant (see X-rays). The patient suffered a fractured pelvis. The conclusion was that the doctor was not in breach of duty and the House of Lords subsequently formulated the Bolam test:

> 'A medical professional is not guilty of negligence if he has acted in accordance with a practice accepted as proper by a responsible body of medical men skilled in that particular art . . . Putting it the other way round, a man is not negligent, if he is acting in accordance with such a practice, merely because there is a body of opinion who would take a contrary view.'[6]

The Bolam test forms the basis of the role of the second opinion appointed doctor (SOAD) when instigating the section 58 procedure of the UK's Mental Health Act 1983.

SOADs were first appointed by the Mental Health Act Commission (MHAC). Originally the Lunacy Commission (1845-1913), then the Board of Control (1913-1959), the MHAC was responsible for ensuring that psychiatry follows the *Mental Health Act Code of Practice* (most recent revision: 2015) in relation to detained patients and issues guidance documents. For Fennell, '...these are forms of 'soft law' [that] seek to develop a system of psychiatric ethics.'[7]

For those detained under the Mental Health Act, the guidance is meant to offer a degree of protection. 'Consent' is not to the fore as detained patients cannot realistically give consent and, again, 'informed' consent is a *non-sequitor* because the person prescribing the electroshock cannot know what will happen.

The 1983 Act followed over a decade of public scandals and inquiries in the UK in a context of almost twenty years of civil rights activism in the US. Inquiries in the UK had been conducted into actions concerning seclusion, restraint, enforced medication and the use of 'emergency' electroshock without anaesthetic in psychiatric hospitals including Ely Hospital, Cardiff, Fairleigh and Whittingham.[8]

The Health and Social Care Act 2008 replaced the Healthcare Commission, the Commission for Social Care Inspection and the Mental Health Act Commission with a single, integrated regulator for health and adult social care – the Care Quality Commission – which began operating on 1 April 2009. Reports from the CQC are available online. For example, a visit to the acute wards and psychiatric intensive care units of Birmingham and Solihull Mental Health NHS Foundation Trust found:

> 'Documentation was poor in some areas. We found some issues with Mental Health Act documentation and recording such as Section 17 paperwork not always showing detail of the conditions of leave or the number of escorts' required and capacity to consent to treatment forms in 43% of the patient records we looked at were not decision specific and did not show how decisions about a patients capacity had been made.' [Sentence exactly as posted] [Updated 1 August 2017][9]

The CQC concluded that 'improvement' was required. A prospective patient in Birmingham is unlikely to read the CQC report and a patient has no control over whether the Trust makes improvements. In a climate of chronic under-staffing, it is not difficult to see why some areas may be neglected. In relation to consent, however, a patient will want to know how likely it is that these failings (by the standards of the CQC) will lead to adverse treatment or effects of treatment. The reader might refer to Assault and Antonin Artaud and Death-making and David Reville for a perspective on why direct harm or adverse effects are likely.

Strictly as probabilities, these calculations are almost impossible. Such calculations would also require on the part of the potential recipient an appreciation of the esoteric world of statistical probability.

Taking 2013 as an example: more than 3 billion people flew on commercial aircraft; there were 81 accidents and 210 fatalities. For UK citizens, the probability of dying in a motor accident is one in 36,512; the chances of dying in a plane crash are one in 3.5m. Aeroplane accidents and terrorist attacks on planes invoke fear for many, a fear that sometimes leads to a refusal to fly. Digital and print media ensure these incidents hit the headlines. The deadliest plane crash in history occurred in 1977 in Tenerife when 583 people were killed after two jumbos collided on the runway. As many people die from heart disease in America every eight hours.[10]

By contrast, death from electroshock rarely hits the headlines (see Opposition and Oprah Winfrey). Between its inception and the 1980s estimates ranged from one to four per cent depending on the age of the recipient, response to anaesthetic, existing medical problems and other factors. Current estimates are closer to one in 100,000. Estimates in the 1980s (taking one in 100 as the most conservative electroshock mortality estimate) made electroshock 365 times more likely to be lethal than car travel and 3,500 times more dangerous than air travel. The figures are best guesses only and hide the question any traveller or electroshock recipient might ask: 'Will *I* be killed?' For psy recipients the question is the obverse of the equally impossible to answer: 'Will this procedure (therapy or drug or electroshock) help *me*?'

Few people understand statistical probabilities but properly constituted consent forms would need to pass tests of comprehensibility as well as readability and one way to make the risk more comprehensible would be to offer risk comparisons as above. Some travellers may conclude journeys merit taking relatively small risks and some potential shock recipients or their guardians may conclude the risk is too high.

In a 2005 study of the use of consent forms, a third of recipients did not feel they had freely consented to electroshock even when they had signed a consent form:

'The proportion who feel they did not freely choose the treatment has actually increased over time. The same themes arise whether the patient had received treatment a year ago or 30 years ago. Neither current nor proposed safeguards for patients are sufficient to ensure informed consent with respect to

ECT, at least in England and Wales.'[11]

The use of written informed consent documents is obligatory in Poland, and reported as 15 per cent in Germany, 44 per cent in Belgium, and 50 per cent in Norway. Written informed consent is mainly obtained from family members in Japan, Thailand and Pakistan and countersigning by a near relative practiced in Saudi Arabia. In Hong Kong, 13 per cent of recipients were judged incapable of giving informed consent.[12]

Examples of consent forms for electroshock are cited by Frank and available online.[13] In fact, factors such as power, legal status, age and the enthusiasm or concern shown by the prescribing psychiatrist make genuinely informed consent an unattainable grail for libertarians. The contextual locus of psy as part of the system of governmentality means that the patient is bound to enter into an unequal contest if she takes the path of resistance; a position reinforced for the prescribing psychiatrist by a professional immersion in the 'safe and effective' rhetoric of electroshock proselytisers (see Marketing and Movies).

One survey of consent with minors given electroshock reveals that less than 20 of 217 cases mentioned consent in published accounts; in the majority of cases the youngsters had refused treatment but shock was nonetheless administered. Parental consent was similarly absent.[14] Baldwin suggests there are more than 230 alternatives. He does not suggest waiting (see X-rays).

For children and adolescents 'consent' is a moot

issue: 'The ability of a pre-teenage child to give *informed* consent is a matter for conjecture.'[15] (original emphasis)

Masson goes further and extends the question of consent to what is known about abuse within talking therapies '... will the patients be given genuine consent even to psychotherapy? Will they be told that the chances of female patients being sexually abused by their therapist are at least 15 per cent?'[16] It is a potential policy that should have given second thoughts to many recipients discussed in this volume.

In the absence of a critical consent form (see Youngsters), perhaps the following may suffice:

> 'You have received a psychiatric diagnosis. This label has no validity. Your consultant prefers to use electroshock in certain situations. The electric shocks will destroy brain cells and will have little beneficial effect in the long term. You may lose many memories – good and bad. You are likely to continue to be medicated with a variety of harmful drugs. There is a chance you will die from the electric shock or anaesthesia.'

Clementine Churchill

The ahistorical tendency of some psychiatric historians to retrospectively inscribe famous folk as depressed would suggest that Winston Churchill (who inscribed himself with the 'Black Dog' of depression) might have been an electroshock candidate. A 1994 study of famous men concludes: 'certain pathological personality characteristics, as well as tendencies towards depression and alcoholism, are causally linked to some kinds of valuable creativity.'[17]

The logical conclusion – that in order to increase creativity someone should become a depressed alcoholic – is not one suggested by psychiatric historians. In 1988 a television discussion programme – *After Dark* – was even trailed as 'Winston Churchill: Hero or Madman?' Creativity notwithstanding (as well as writing the four volume *A History of the English Speaking Peoples,* Churchill was a fine painter) Churchill's role as British Prime Minister 1940-1945 spared him electroshock.

But, at the outbreak of World War I, pregnant and left alone by her husband to look after two small children and her neurasthenic mother, Clementine Churchill had attempted self-harm. When her two-year-old daughter Marigold died of septicaemia in 1921, she collapsed. Forty years later, after supporting her husband's topsy-turvy political career, in early October, 1962, she was inscribed with depression, sedated and admitted to Westminster Hospital, and electroshocked.

Anthony Montague Browne, Winston's private secretary from 1952 (and, as it happens the father of Justin Welby, Archbishop of Canterbury) until his employer's death remembered that the shock treatment was for 'a (so-called) chemical imbalance in her brain.'

Clementine was still in the hospital when, during the night of October 19-20, 1962 her daughter Diana who had also been receiving electroshock, took an overdose of sleeping pills and was found dead on the bedroom floor of her Belgravia flat by her housekeeper.

Notwithstanding her indefatigable support for her husband, Clementine frequently took to her bed, sometimes for a day or two, perhaps as a defence against the demands of her challenging spouse. In 1963, she was again hospitalized and given electroshock. After Winston's death her nervous complaints largely disappeared.[18]

Death-making
and David Reville

Wolf Wolfensberger coined the term 'Death-making' to refer to human service practices causing spiritual or physical harm (including hastening death) to their recipients.[1]

Notably, the fifth edition of the *Diagnostic and Statistical Manual of Mental Disorders* (*DSM-5*) lists neuroleptic-induced brain disorders such as tardive dyskinesia as 'mental disorders' rather than iatrogenic assaults, a specific denial of the death-making inherent in taking psychiatric drugs. Similarly, disorders of memory caused by electroshock do not appear as amnesia of known origin.

Almost all formal interventions carried out by human services produce 'wounds' of one type or another. For Wolfensberger the wounds include any action that removes a person from valued and normative settings and relationships. For example, a person might be *rejected* or *excluded* (from a family, school, valued neighbourhood or activity) 'for their own good'.

A psychological assessment might here suggest transfer to a specialist environment, for example, a centre for those inscribed as anorexic or eating disordered. Once placed elsewhere a person might be quickly *moved* (often *without explanation*) thus *losing any new relationships* in the service setting where the person is now *isolated* and *congregated* with other service recipients (who may only have in common the fact that their families and society finds them obnoxious and difficult to get on with, or criminalizes them or inscribes them as disabled, disordered or disturbed).

Once moved and inscribed people will *lack security and control*. They will be *marked* – inscribed and re-inscribed with psy-terminology (frequently via psychometric testing) that shifts their identity onto an 'abnormal' or 'mentally ill' spectrum and leads to *confusion* concerning what they need (see Inscription and Insulin coma). It can, for example, be assumed that a lonely, frightened child 'needs' drugs rather than a safe place with caring others or it might be taken for granted that a wheelchair user is experiencing other physical difficulties.

Vagaries of the benefits system mean that a further wound for those institutionalised is *becoming poorer*. Service recipients may also be *blamed* for resistance to treatment, *subject to humiliating case conferences*, *invaded* (for example with injections of PRN medication) *without consent, referred to other agencies without consent, denied help* and *given aversive or useless 'treatments.'*

Beyond these entirely legal interventions, service recipients may be *abused* in institutions and will, invariably, be *subject to the gaze*.[2]

The potentially harmful nature of service interventions means that psy professionals are likely to be involved in death-making, at least as bystanders (see; Bystanders and Bud Powell). Additionally, some practitioners set out to harm, though the majority espouse more charitable motivations. Declaring their essential beneficence via professional codes of conduct, professions such as nursing or clinical psychology would vehemently deny their role in death-making.

Wolfensberger suggests, however, that killing of the spirit is everyday practice for many professionals, even those involved in non-physical interventions like counselling; patients most often need changes to their *circumstances* not technicalised conversations. A patient who doesn't change may be blamed by the therapist for a 'lack of motivation' or may self-blame with a consequent reduction in spirit.

For clients and patients of counsellors and other therapists the sense of double failure (as person and patient) is made more likely by regular media exaggeration of the success of interventions such as Cognitive Behaviour Therapy (CBT). Wolfensberger's position echoes that of the sociologist, Gruenberg, who coined the term 'the social breakdown syndrome' as a way of describing the institutionally produced emotional impact on psychiatric patients.[3]

Potential death-making and 'sacrifice' in the name of learning and 'progress' has long been a medical tradition, possibly from the first time a Neolithic healer self-administered a potential herbal remedy. For centuries the 'sacrifice' has been largely that of patients whose physicians try out experimental procedures, sometimes as a last resort. Most bodily fluids have been theorised about and reduced or modified. Similarly, most organs in the body – from the liver to the brain via the spleen – have been implicated in the experience of madness and operated on or removed.

In 1872 Hegar, professor of obstetrics at Freiburg, carried out the first ovariotomy. The procedure was soon regarded as a cure for hysteria. By the 1890s, male castration was seen as the cure for criminality. In both cases the destruction of healthy organs was based on theoretical supposition, a precursor to the century of destruction of brain matter with dubious justification that was to follow.

Paul Weindling sees this surgical interventionism as laying the basis for extensive eugenic programmes – hereditists could argue that even if ovariotomy and castration did not cure the patient, the surgery prevented genetic transmission of disease to the next generation. Hegar feared a society dominated by the degenerate masses more concerned with individual pleasure seeking than committed to the fate of society as a whole.

In 1899, the industrialist and social Darwinist Friedrich Kruup funded the Jena prize for a scientific answer to the question: 'What can we learn from the principles of evolution for the development of laws and states?' The closing date was 1 December 1902. The winning entrant, Shallmayer, used Weismann's theories of selectionist biology to formulate a code of 'generative ethics' – the 'unfit' would be prevented from reproducing. The degenerative included '... the insane, the feeble-minded, and the alcoholic, those infected by

TB and VD, and criminals. '[4]

Over the following years, the theories of Hegar and of Shallmayer became part of the justificatory rhetoric for forced sterilization in many industrialized countries including the US and Germany. In the late 1930s the theory of degeneration with its blend of biology and implications for state welfare and economic health allowed literal death-making to take place in psychiatric hospitals in Germany.

Hitler's first declarations against the weak, whose lives were 'burdensome' for the state had been at the Nuremberg Party rally of 1929. After he gained power there was a relentless progression to the 'final solution' in which psychiatry would be a forerunner: 'While 'euthanasia' of the supposedly incurable was supported and legitimised by Hitler ... medical experts took a crucial role in its administration ... The victims were primarily children of under three years of age, diagnosed as mentally retarded or congenitally malformed, and the mentally ill.'[5]

A group including Phillippe Bouhler, Victor Brack (Hitler's physician) and the paediatricians Wentzler and Catel initiated killing under the auspices of the 'Reich Committee for the Scientific Registration of Serious Hereditary and Congenital Illnesses.'

In October 1939, Hitler enabled Bouhler and Brandt to begin *Gnatentod* (mercy killing) of patients judged incurable. The psychiatric team responsible for implementing *Gnatentod* was soon joined by an advocate of insulin shock, Nitsche. In December 1939, Jewish and Polish patients from Meseritz-Obrawalde were killed by a strong sedative (in woods near to the hospital). Staff tried gassing patients as a more efficient method of killing and in June 1940 the gassing of Jewish patients began.

Far from being bystanders in the process of extermination, psychiatric staff were part of the Nazi machinery. Robert Lifton reveals that by 1933 the majority of German psychiatrists were already members of the SS having joined on ideological grounds; the concept of a 'dilution' of Aryanism fitted well with existing psy theories of 'degeneration.'[6]

The first gas chambers were constructed in German hospitals. The aim was to kill via carbon monoxide or starvation incarcerated patients inscribed as psychotic and children said to have genetic illnesses. Robert Proctor refers to the 'banality' of the procedure noting that: 'In 1941 the psychiatric institution of Hadamar celebrated the cremation of its ten-thousandth patient in a special ceremony, where everyone in attendance – secretaries, nurses and psychiatrists – received a bottle of beer for the occasion.'[7]

That same year, Eugen Fischer (who lived on for over 20 years after the war), the co-director of the Kaiser Wilhelm Institute for Archaeology, declared Bolsheviks and Jews to be a distinct degenerative species. And once an entire race is no longer considered human, the way is opened up for members to be herded up and slaughtered.[8]

Death wasn't inevitable but psychiatrically induced torment was a certainty. In his 'Expression of gratitude' to psychiatric survivor and activist Dorothea Buck,

41

Peter Lehmann says: 'Dorothea was a victim of forced sterilization during the Nazi era. Beside this mutilation, she also suffered buckets of cold water poured over her head, lengthy baths in a tub covered with canvas, cold wet sheets, cardiazol-, insulin- and electro-shock, injections of paraldehyde and she witnessed the effects of neuroleptics in her fellow patients (she also uses the name Sophie Zerchin, rearranging the letters of the German word for 'schizophrenia.')'[9]

For some, it may seem extreme to connect Nazi Germany with the psy professions. For historians the links are indissoluble. Ideologically they are linked through the idea that people can be inferior/superior to each other in skills and genetically determined attributes. The search for genetic origins of Aryanism mirrors that for the genetic origins (or predisposition) to schizophrenia.

Both systems define (*pace* Foucault) normality by default through definitions of degeneration/ abnormality/madness/disease. A paradox here is that, for thirty years following the Second World War, the notional average European family (an invention) had 2.2 children. For fin de siècle German eugenicists, however, using contraception to limit a family to two children was a sign of counter-Nationalist feeling and degeneracy; the eugenicist position was an explicit attempt to keep the frau chained.

Beyond theory and philosophy, both systems have been dominated by a death-making culture and a system of self-promotion based on public fear – in much the same way that the Nazis promised freedom from debt and war in the 1920s, psychiatry has, for two hundred years, made an (unfulfilled) promise of freeing us from madness and dangerously mad citizens.

Like Nazism, psychiatry expands its list of degenerates. For the Nazis, the categorization encompassed first the psychotic, then children with disabilities, then Bolsheviks and Jews, finally Gypsies. For psychiatry, an ever expanding classification system (from 112 diagnoses in *DSM-I* to 365 in *DSM-5* over 60 years later) has, since the *DSM-III* of 1980, potentially included us all.

Any totalitarian system requires a justificatory ideology and the ideologies of Nazism and psychiatry can appear uncomfortably close. Contemporary supporters of the screening of children, inscription, medication and electroshock, bolstered by theories of hereditary psychiatric disorder and notions of 'acceptable' conduct, would contest any attempt to equate their principles with what has become circumscribed as 'Nazi ideology'.

The assumed inevitability of inheriting madness and criminal traits was, however, commonplace by the end of the nineteenth century (see Normality and Novels). Between 1900 and 1939, British eugenicists included psychologists Burt, Spearman and Pearson (holder of the inaugural Galton chair in eugenics at University College, London). Writing on Beyondism, the eugenics movement he founded, the US psychologist Cattell claimed;

'The vast majority of humans on the planet are

'obsolete' and… the earth will be choked with the more primitive forerunners unless a way is found to eliminate them…Clarity of discussion…would be greatly aided if genocide were reserved for a literal killing off of all living members of a people…and genthanasia for what has been above called 'phasing out,' in which a moribund culture is ended, by educational and birth control measures.'[10]

Cattell was writing just over sixty years ago, some 27 years *after* the Holocaust. Intellectuals such as the socialist Webbs, Havelock Ellis and George Bernard Shaw as well as the Blackshirts of Oswald Moseley were all eugenicist. Sociologists are likely to see notions of unbounded 'spectrum disorders' and 'family histories' of madness as related to the eugenic thrust of the first half of the last century.

'Risk' of inheritance of certain so called disorders is now a standard assumption in psychiatry and underlies UK protocols for tests and scans of potentially Down's Syndrome foetuses carried out in ante-natal clinics. In combination with the idea of a disorder spectrum and the desirability of 'health' (for the purposes here defined as a comfortable life and the absence of debilitating illness) screening foetuses is equivalent to screening children and, where deemed necessary, inscribing then prescribing to those children.

David Reville
As noted in Bystanders and Bud Powell, the silence from professionals on practices such as electroshock

can be deafening; over thirty years less than a dozen articles in the monthly UK Division of Clinical Psychology newsletter, *Clinical Psychology Forum,* have examined the ethics or harmful consequences of electroshock. Survivors and activists rather than psy professionals form the bed-rock of the electroshock protest community, a community that interlinks with numerous other survivor groups. Many professional and academic writers take particular critical positions.

For example, criticism can come through the lens of feminism or gender-politics. Other critique can be more abstruse; post-structuralism can be combined with Marxist theory and psycho-analysis to dizzying effect. For many survivor groups, however, protest stems from physical harm and a sense of betrayal; it might be worth noting that qualifying medical students no longer pledge to 'First do no harm'.

David Reville, was born in Brantford, Ontario. After graduating from Brantford Collegiate Institute in 1961, he attended Trinity College at the University of Toronto, going on to law school. It was expected that he would follow the career path of his father, an Ontario judge. Instead, Reville attempted to kill himself during his law studies. After institutionalization in a psychiatric hospital, he was inscribed with manic depression and given electroshock. On release, he became a crusader for mental health reform.

In 1993, he co-founded Mad Pride, a mass movement of the users and recipients of mental health services, former users, and their allies. The organization began as a response to local community prejudices towards people with a psychiatric history living in boarding homes in the Parkdale area of Toronto, Canada. A similar movement began around the same time in the UK. By the late 1990s, events were being organized under the Mad Pride name in England, Australia, South Africa and the United States. According to Mind Freedom International, a United States mental health advocacy organization, events now draw thousands of participants.[11]

Evidence and Electrocution

Synonyms for the word evident include: obvious, apparent, noticeable, conspicuous, visible, perceivable, perceptible, observable, clear, crystal clear, clear-cut, writ large, plain, manifest.

For science and scientism (the appearance of being scientific), the word evidence means something different. Evidence is said to be found when certain statistical criteria are met. Thus, it may be obvious that electrocuting a person is harmful but, if such assault is subjected to statistical analysis it might be shown that for a proportion of people electrocution is regarded as helpful.

In the domain of psy, there is not that much research necessary. We know what hurts people: exploitation, humiliation, cruelty, inflexible ideologies, torture, starvation, and the substitution of hate for love. We know that electrocution is very dangerous. The research endeavour is, however, driven by the desire for cultural capital and financial reward as much as a desire for understanding.

A high proportion of evidence in the field of human science is actually gathered via analogy. As experimentation on human subjects is bounded by ethical restrictions, animal subjects or virtual science is used. In research on new cancer drugs, for example, mice are classic subjects. This spares immediate harm to potential human subjects and recipients of anti-cancer agents but raises questions including the ethics of animal experimentation and the accuracy of the animal-human analogy.

For many, it is ethically acceptable to experiment on dogs, mice, rabbits and so on if the avoidance of human suffering is the goal. Rabbits blinded by research designed to decrease the chances of shampoo stinging a child's eyes are an acceptable by-product of a moral research enterprise (see Marketing and Movies).

It may seem self-evident that passing electric current through the brain is harmful, but evidence of harm is still demanded by those advocating electroshock as a treatment. As a wide age range of people across the world receive electroshock after a variety of psychiatric inscriptions (diagnoses) and prescriptions there is no need for analogous animal studies on outcome. Evidence is available direct from recipients via interview, from data on morbidity and, indirectly, via psychometrics.

An immediate challenge to such evidence gathering is the lack of validity of psychiatric diagnoses (see Inscription and Insulin coma). A label with no construct validity (for example, there is no *a priori* reason for clustering early morning waking with tearfulness when seeking to label someone depressed) presents researchers with even more difficulty if it is used differently by two or more different diagnosticians and thus lacks reliability.

We can't say with any confidence that electroshock

is effective for depression, for example, if depression is an invalid and unreliable construct and research concerning those labelled depressed thus involves a disparate rather than homogeneous group.

For the patients of clinical psychologists working in services with a high proportion of older people assessments of, for example, 'dementia vs depression' will have important consequences. Older women are the largest group receiving electroshock which has been described as the 'treatment of choice' for people over 60 deemed depressed. Clinical psychologists working in services for older people frequently offer therapeutic alternatives to electrocution but the zeitgeist is such that the majority of persons over the age of 60 inscribed as depressed will receive drug treatment or electroshock rather than kindly comfort from a psy professional.

Evidence for the prevalence of electroshock is as difficult to obtain as research studies on outcome – see Research and Robeson. Data on the practice of electroshock in the UK reveals widely varying use between NHS administrative regions. Shock data were routinely collected by the National Health Service until 1991, when specific electroshock reporting was replaced by Hospital Episode Statistics, considered to significantly under-report electroshock activity. In a survey conducted that year, two authorities, Mid-Staffordshire and Herefordshire, used very little while others in the same West Midlands region electroshocked more than one in ten psychiatric admissions.

Typically about two-thirds of recipients were women. In Great Yarmouth and Waveney less than one in a hundred admissions were electroshocked; in the adjacent East Suffolk, one in five admissions were recipients.[1]

Standards and practice vary remarkably, not only between different countries but also within them and even within individual centres; there has been an 18-fold difference in use of electroshock between 11 general adult psychiatric teams within a single Edinburgh teaching hospital. Further, during 2000–2001, the Mental Health Act Commission reported that there were substantial departures from best policy, practice or training in a fifth of 230 facilities they surveyed in England and Wales.[2]

To attempt to improve quality control of electroshock administration, the Royal Colleges of Psychiatrists, Anaesthetists and Nursing launched the ECT Accreditation Service (ECTAS) in May 2003. Membership of ECTAS is voluntary. ECTAS surveyed mental health trusts that had used electroshock between September 2004 and February 2006. The protocol included a questionnaire for recipients of whom 72 per cent said the intervention had been helpful, 20 per cent that it had had no effect, five per cent that they would not want it again and 14 per cent that it had changed or saved their lives.[3]

The incidence of electroshock was assessed in 56 clinics over three months in England in 2006 (private clinics were excluded). Compared with 1999 and 2002 the number of clinics providing electroshock and the number of patients receiving it had declined (down to an estimated 1,276) of whom a higher proportion (30%) received electroshock as involuntary patients under the Mental Health Act.[4]

It is still used in England without national auditing. A 2017 study used Freedom of Information Act requests to gather information from 56 National Health Service Trusts on usage, demographics, consent, and adherence to the guidelines of the National Institute of Clinical Excellence (NICE) and to the Mental Health Act of which 32 trusts provided usable information. The study concluded that the number of people currently receiving electroshock in England annually is between 2,100 and 2,700 and:

'There was a 12- fold difference between the Trusts with the highest and lowest usage rates per capita. Most recipients are still women (66%) and over 60 (56%). More than a third (39%) is given without consent, with 30% of Trusts not adhering to mental health legislation concerning second opinions. At least 44% were not using validated measures of efficacy, and at least 33% failed to do so for adverse effects. Only four provided any actual data for positive outcomes or adverse effects. None provided any data on efficacy beyond the end of treatment. An investigation into why ECT is still administered excessively to older people and women seems long overdue.'[5]

For many anti-electroshock campaigners the question

of why it is used at all – with men or women – is more pertinent. Some potential answers are provided in this volume (see Vested interest and Vaslav Nijinsky and Women).

Any answer is itself governed by self-interest: an individualistic turn suggests it is 'self-evident' that researchers carry out electroshock for money, publication and cultural capital, psychiatrists prescribe it for money and a desire to do something for patients who are distressed, frustrated by the psychiatrist's efforts and frustrating to the professionals involved, and patients want it because changing their relationships or other circumstances may be as impossible as changing or accepting their past histories – even assuming their past histories matter. For some, it may be self-evident that parents want it for their children as a form of punishment whilst others see parents as advocating a 'life and family saving' intervention, a claim also made on behalf of parents who seek inscriptions of ADHD for their off-spring in order to access Ritalin to give the family a little peace.[6]

Introducing the Psy-complex and its interventions into a family may well change family life. There is, however, no evidence that electroshock is a life saver. In a study comparing suicidal people who had been electroshocked with a group who hadn't Avery and Winokur found, '... treatment was not shown to affect the suicide rate.'[7] Peter Breggin concludes: 'Overall, there is little or nothing in the literature to suggest that ECT ameliorates suicide whereas a significant body of literature confirms that it does not.'[8]

Again, this is, to an extent, self-evident. Numerous people who have received electroshock have gone on to kill themselves just as numerous people who take anti-depressants go on to take over-doses. Curative or not for some, it cannot be claimed that electroshock or psychopharmacology prevent suicide.

I have suggested elsewhere that one potential explanation for a psychiatrist's use of electroshock is hatred of women – particularly older women.[9] The view is quickly dismissed by those who feels accused – as if, in a misogynist culture professionals can move beyond the zeitgeist. Curiously, however, a 45-year-old survey by Pallis and Stoffelmayr did show that psychiatrists who favour physical interventions tend to hold conservative social values and are 'tough-minded.'[10]

Many activists and critics regard survivor accounts of electroshock's legacy of personal harm as sufficient evidence; many others have sought out scientific research to support their position. Leonard Roy Frank (1932-2015) was one such psychiatric survivor and activist in the patients' rights movement. In 1962, he was committed to a psychiatric hospital after being inscribed as 'paranoid schizophrenic' and given 50 insulin coma treatments and 35 electroshock sessions.

He joined the staff of 'Madness Network News,' and in December 1973, with Wade Hudson founded Network Against Psychiatric Assault (NAPA), a patients' and survivors' advocacy group and inspiration for the formation of MindFreedom. His most famous book, *The History of Shock Treatment*, published in 1978, was the most detailed history of electroshock to that point. For Frank it is self-evident that electric shocks to the head are dangerous. As he says:

'The nature of the human brain and that of electricity are no different today than they were more than 50 years ago.... Whatever may be the ameliorating factors of the newer delivery techniques, when a convulsogenic dose of electricity is applied to the brain, there is going to be a certain amount of brain damage ... the more current applied, the more amnesia and brain damage.' [11]

Peter Breggin compares electroshock with closed head injury and cites McClelland and colleagues' description of the post concussive syndrome: 'somatic symptoms (headaches, dizziness, fatigability) accompanied by psychological symptoms (memory and concentration difficulties, irritability, emotional lability, depression and anxiety).' [12]

Friedberg published the first review of brain damage caused by electroshock, a study that was not cited in the 1990 APA Task force report (see Vested interest and Vaslav Nijinsky). [13] Babayan suggested there was ' .. convincing proof ... pointing to grave changes in the central nervous system, the nerve cells, the glial-tissue apparatus ...' [14] Like Breggin, Babayan compares electroshock to lobotomy. Although he states: 'There has been contradictory evidence of ECT damage in brain-scan studies ...,' [15] like Babayan Breggin finally called for a ban: 'If ordinary medical ethics were applied to psychiatry, based on nothing more than the original large-animal studies, shock treatment would be prohibited.'[16]

Due to the relatively large number of deaths following electroshock in the first decades, autopsy evidence is available. It reveals visible pathology arising from brain trauma.[17] This seems of little concern to shock advocates who see a need for cell damage to ensure the required loss of memory or to those who quote contrasting evidence from studies showing an absence of brain damage.

Like inscription itself the field is widening: Bipolar disorder and Bipolar II disorder were first included in the *Diagnostic and Statistical Manual* in 1980 (*DSM-III*) and 1994 (*DSM-IV*) respectively. A chapter in *The Bipolar Book: History, Neurobiology and Treatment* is devoted to electroshock.[18] The authors point out that searching PubMed for 'bipolar disorder electroconvulsive therapy' returns more than 1,000 citations and agree with a 1994 review study, the FDA and NICE that electroshock should be a treatment option for mania.[19]

Electrocution

After killing a spectator in 1902 at the Forepaugh Circus, Topsy (a female Asian elephant born around 1875) was sold to Coney Island's Sea Lion Park (see front cover illustration). When Sea Lion was leased out at the end of the 1902 season and redeveloped into Luna Park, Topsy's owners planned to hang her at the park in a public spectacle but were stopped by the *American Society for the Prevention of Cruelty to*

Animals. Instead, on January 4 1903, in front of a small crowd of invited reporters and guests Topsy was fed poison, electrocuted, and strangled, the electrocution ultimately killing her. Amongst the press that day was a crew from the *Edison Manufacturing* movie company. Their film of the electrocution part was released to be viewed in coin-operated kinetoscopes under the title *Electrocuting an Elephant.*[20]

I have twice been electrocuted. The first time, on a building site in my teens, I touched the bare live cable on a faulty electric drill. Earthed via rubber soles on a pair of sturdy boots, I felt a powerful jolt to my arm – and nothing more. It was painful for a few seconds, and I remained alert enough to employ at least one Anglo-Saxon expletive. Some 30 years later, I managed to prod a screwdriver into a live electric socket. This time, minus any rubber soles, my body jerked backwards and I awoke after a few seconds of unconsciousness having hit the edge of the kitchen table with some force; electrocution is not something to take lightly.

The history and current practice of electroshock is marked by a combination of serious intent and a flexible (critics might suggest cavalier) approach to electrocution. Cerletti, who had worked with Franz Nissl, neuropathologist and neuro-anatomist in Heidelberg, wanted to integrate his results from histopathology with the biological study of emotions. Bini, under Cerletti's instruction, built the first electro-shock apparatus as a tool for research.

Following Nyirö's theory about the impossibility of schizophrenia and epilepsy co-existing, Cerletti dedicated himself to researching easier and less toxic ways than metrazol to cause epileptic convulsions. For several years, in Genoa, he carried out experimental studies of epilepsy, provoking epileptic seizures in animals (in particular in dogs) via electrocution. He used domestic electricity (alternating current at 125 volts) for a fraction of a second, with two electrodes, one placed in the mouth and the other in the rectum.

Numerous experiments with human subjects were performed over a period of two months: according to the different electric resistance, these employed currents with intensities between 300 and 600 mA, potential differences between 80 and 115 volts, and durations of 0.5 - 0.7 seconds.[21]

Accounts differ concerning the first experimental shocks with Enrico X (see History and Hemingway). Observing pigs at the slaughterhouse Cerletti and Bini had learned that there was a wide margin between the charge needed to shock (120 volts) and a fatal dose (400 volts). Passive, and with his head shaven, Enrico X lay on a bed and had two electrodes attached to his temples. He was provided with a gauze-wrapped gum pipe to bite on. For Norman Endler: 'Bini adjusted the equipment to 110 volts and three quarters of a second, and Felici clicked the switch.'[22]

Using Cerletti and Bini's original publication Aruta suggests that the first shock was at 80 volts for a quarter of a second followed by another at the same voltage for half a second ten minutes later. A third dose for three quarters of a second also failed to produce the required convulsion. A week later Bini applied 92 volts for half a second and Enrico X entered history as the first inscribed recipient of an electrically induced fit.[23]

As evidence of electrocution original source material is, however, unreliable. According to Roberta Passione, who has made a study of Lucio Bini's notebooks, the events outlined by their student Accornero are a fiction.[24] For Aruta, the reported events '... constitute an 'electro-shock novel' which was authored by the self-celebrating Cerletti through the control he exercised over what his students could report.' She goes on: 'It is a self-fashioned heroic science narrative' and quotes Passione in saying the story, '... crosses the border of myth.'[25]

Bini patented the machine and exported it around the world; the economic gain was considerable. Various models were developed and successfully marketed, including the portable one held in the *Museo di Storia della Medicina della Sapienza* at the University of Rome, where, in 2011 an exhibition was organized around the Bini–Cerletti apparatus. The exhibition's director described the machine (in the context of 1930s Fascist Italy) as, '... at one and the same time a blessing, a hope, a lie, and a profitable commercial product.' [26]

Most modern electroshock devices deliver a brief-pulse current, which is thought to cause fewer cognitive effects than the sine-wave currents originally used. A small minority of psychiatrists in the US still use sine-wave stimuli. Sine-wave is no longer used in the UK or Ireland. Typically, the electrical stimulus used is about 800 milliamps and has up to several hundred watts. The current flows for between one and six seconds.

In the US, shock devices are manufactured by two companies, Somatics, which is owned by psychiatrists Richard Abrams and Conrad Swartz, and Mecta (see Vested interest and Vaslav Nijinsky). In the UK, the market for shock devices is monopolized by Ectron Ltd, founded in 1950 by psychiatrist Robert Russell. Ectron also markets the DuoMagXT rTMS system for the 'clinical treatment of depression.'[27]

'Electrocution' is not a term preferred by advocates of electroshock. Research has consistently shown that it is the charge rather than the convulsion that produces the necessary brain damage and mood effect yet the trope 'therapy' remains the usual nomenclature even amongst activists who join 'ECT' chat groups or 'ECT' protest groups on the Internet. From Bini and Cerletti to contemporary practitioners, however, electrocution is what is practised though with less danger of bone breakages (see X-rays).

New praxis requires less disturbing imagery and a more marketable lexis. Enter magnetic seizure therapy (MST), promoted by Sarah Lisanby, MD, chief of the division of brain stimulation and therapeutic modulation at Columbia University. Lisanby uses the trope of safety as part of MST's appeal: 'We want to take advantage of the efficacy of ECT but try to make it more available by making it safer.' Tim Jarvis (see Opposition and Oprah Winfrey) concurs, '... radical – and exciting for the treatment-resistant depressed – are brain implants that work like pacemakers to keep a lagging neural area up to speed.'

The implants transmit a constant low-voltage

current to an area called the subgenual cingulate region, or Brodmann area 25 (deep brain stimulation; DBS).[28]

Positioning magnetically-induced seizures as 'stimulation' and electrocution as safe, benign and even reparative adds to the mystique. Images of a convulsing Jack Nicholson in *One Flew Over the Cuckoo's Nest* can be consigned to the dustbin of an un-enlightened past.

Fits and
Frances Farmer

During electroshock, an electric current is passed briefly through the brain, via electrodes applied to the scalp, to induce generalised seizure activity.[1] The treatment is usually bilateral (electrodes placed on both temples), though this varies. The person being shocked is anaesthetised; muscle relaxants are given to prevent spasms.

This also varies (see below): 'unmodified' shock – without anaesthesia, with consequent skeletal fractures – is practised in Africa, Turkey, Russia, China and some other countries. Melinda James, an electroshock survivor, has also questioned the efficacy of the anaesthesia in modified shock:

'The drug they give to avoid bones breaking is NOT a muscle relaxant. It is a muscle paralyser. It paralyses all the muscles. You cannot blink your eyes, you cannot breathe. I know because one time or maybe more (I only remember one) they did not give me enough of the anaesthetic, and I was not asleep. I could not tell them I was fully conscious - could not move, could not blink my eyes. I saw the doctor leaning over me with the electrodes. Then I was knocked out by the shock. Fully conscious, but paralysed, it felt like someone had bashed my head in with a hammer.'[2]

In the UK, it is recommended that electroshock is given twice a week up to a maximum of six weeks; again, this varies (see below). Repeated treatments induce molecular and cellular changes in the brain, characterised by psychiatrist Peter Breggin as 'brain damage' and an 'electrical lobotomy'.[3,4] Weiner agrees, noting that an electroencephalogram (EEG) will detect brain injury following unilateral shock.[5] Neurologists Symonds and Sament compare the cerebral damage of the practice to head injury.[6,7] Similarly, McClelland sees post-shock changes as identical to classic signs of frontal lobe damage.[8]

Although Cerletti and Bini were convinced by the need to invoke epileptiform seizures in keeping with Julius Nyirö's theory concerning schizophrenia (see; History and Hemingway), it has long since been accepted that it is the extent and force of electric shock that produce the effect. This has been directly linked to the destruction of cerebral matter. In short the greater the shock, the more brain damage and the greater loss of memory and concomitant (temporary) change in mood.

Fits are not needed and promotional campaigns on You-tube contrast the frightening scenes of convulsions in the past with relatively mild visible external effects today. The presenter of one brief clip states that there is poor evidence for shock's effectiveness in schizophrenia implying, by default, that it is effective for those she calls depressed. She maintains the myth of the importance of convulsion by referring to 'seizure.'[9]

Cameron summarises the now seventy year old rejection of the convulsion hypothesis: For Wilcox - a decade after Cerletti and Bini's first experimentation (see; History and Hemingway) – electrical stimulation of the brain was all that was necessary to produce an 'anti-depressant effect.'[10]

Wilcox's term 'electrostimulation' could be seen as prescient given the current vogue for repetitive transcranial magnetic stimulation (rTMS see Zealotry and Zelda Fitzgerald), a procedure that has already moved from the clinic and was used by the US team at the 2018 winter Olympics. Grand mal seizures of the required strength only needed enough electricity to induce them rather than the charge produced by the mass-produced Cerletti-Bini device. Thus 'adequate' convulsions, '... could be induced with lower dosages of electricity' than found in the Cerletti-Bini machines. Ergo, 'Cerletti and Bini's device ... was not an *electroconvulsive* device, but an electroshock device.'[11]

To be sure, as already acknowledged by review papers in the 1940s, the lower dosage produced brain damage and memory loss, but it was – and remains – the electric shock rather than the convulsion that leads to these changes.[12,13,14] As noted in X-rays, convulsions lead to bone breakages but the notorious 'fit' has never had a real impact on any desired outcomes. These findings are further complicated by research that consistently shows that 'sham' (or placebo) electroshock has the same effects in terms of mood as real electroshock – neither the convulsion *nor* the charge is necessary (see Evidence and Electrocution).

Competition within the industry now highlights the absence of fits and in some cases electricity itself as a way of selling 'safer' interventions. Working for Brainstorm, the Stanford Laboratory for Brain Health Innovation and Entrepreneurship ('...the first of its kind.'), a group of psychiatric researchers claim to be, '... applying the biopsychosocial model of disease to tackle problems on the systems level.'

As a business enterprise Brainstorm has no interest in tackling the problem at the level of capitalism. The first three authors are founders of Brainstorm while Nagpal and McKenzie are junior fellows. A note states: 'Dr. Chaudhary, Dr. Aragam, Ms. Nagpal, Ms. McKenzie, and Ms. Chen report no conflicts of interest concerning the subject matter of this article.' Brainstorm claims to be, '... the world's first academic laboratory dedicated to transforming brain health through entrepreneurship.'[15]

Is any of this necessary? Many cultures don't use drugs or electroshock to change consciousness. Popular though stories of South American and Pacific Islander peoples ingesting hallucinogens may be, chanting, singing and drumming alone have been used for centuries in healing ceremonies. Anyone who listens to Charlie Watts, Jim Keltner or the Burundi drummers on Joni Mitchell's *Hissing of Summer Lawns* will soon understand the power of rhythm.

Neher showed electroencephalogram changes in people listening to drum beats[16] and Jilek demonstrated that rhythmic drumming in indigenous

North American healing ceremonies produced adrenaline secretion (as did fasting; another reason that self-starvation inscribed as anorexia is so difficult to give up. The only equivalent is to fall in love).[17]

Fuller Torrey notes that these changes are the equivalent of trance-states induced at rock concerts that may serve as a kind of psychotherapy for both the teenagers at the concert and parents, '...who enjoy a quiet house for the evening': a benignly conservative view of dual happy parenting that is, in itself, rooted in myth.[18]

The complexities of inscription and prescription are part of the package – a kind of unstated rhetoric that are, in themselves, part of the expert dance. Within a hierarchical culture of expertise, the power to electrocute others seems irresistible. There are alternatives – drumming may feel addictive, but there are few adverse effects (notwithstanding the scene in *Love Actually* where Liam Neeson is driven to distraction by his drum-apprentice step-son).

Frances Farmer

By 1942, the actress Frances Farmer had appeared in fourteen films. Amongst others she had co-starred with Cary Grant and Bing Crosby. In that year, her reportedly erratic conduct was made public. After several arrests and committals to psychiatric institutions, Farmer was inscribed with manic depressive psychosis and paranoid schizophrenia. At the request of her mother, she was relocated from Los Angeles to Western State Hospital in her home state of Washington. She was given insulin coma therapy and electroshock and was compulsorily incarcerated between 1945 and 1950.

In her posthumously published autobiography *Will There Really Be a Morning?* Farmer talks of being brutalized and mistreated in numerous ways including being forced to eat her own faeces and act as a sex slave for male doctors and orderlies. Farmer recounted her stay in the state asylum as 'unbearable terror':

> 'I was raped by orderlies, gnawed on by rats and poisoned by tainted food. I was chained in padded cells, strapped into strait-jackets and half-drowned in ice baths.'[19]

She died in 1970.

Farmer's life and mythology have been pursued through film, on the stage and in music. Jessica Lange played her in the 1982 film, *Frances* and Sheila McLaughlin directed and co-wrote, with novelist Lynne Tillman, the 1984 film *Committed*. Nirvana are one of several bands to reference her. *In Utero* features 'Frances Farmer Will Have Her Revenge on Seattle' by Kurt Cobain.

Governmentality
and Gene Tierney

Samuel Bentham was working as an overseer in Krichev (white Russia, now Belarus) when visited by his brother, Jeremy, in the late 1780s. His suggestion – a circular building as the hub of a larger factory where unskilled workers could be observed by a few managers – was taken up by Jeremy Bentham as a model for prisons.

Named the *panopticon*, the concept included the notion that prisoners would not know when their cell was being watched and would begin to monitor each other to ensure their own cell group wasn't punished. Bentham described the panopticon as 'a new mode of obtaining power of mind over mind.'[1]

Despite promises from the government at the time, Bentham's prison was never built. Bentham found a form of revenge for the failure of both English and French administrations to take up his ideas. He claimed that University College, London would be a major beneficiary if his cadaver was mummified, stuffed and put on display. He still sits at his desk in a glass case (an auto-icon), in full view of visitors, a life mask on his face, pen in mummified hand. He had purchased a one hundredth share in UCL's foundation – for one pound.

The panoptical principle, however, of control via a

system of observance where the watched don't know when they are being watched is now commonplace. CCTV cameras are present in numerous public spaces and when speaking to companies by phone both caller and recipient are informed they are being recorded 'for training purposes.'

Governmentality is 'the ensemble formed by institutions, procedures, analyses and reflections, the calculations and tactics, that allow the exercise of this very specific albeit complex form of power, which has its target population'.[2] One aspect of governmentality is the inscription of the self.

The gaze of psy has been fundamental to this inscription. Rose suggests the origins of observational psy praxis can be traced to the work of, among others, Darwin, Sully and Stanley Hall.[3] All three observed and documented infants and drew parents into a disciplinary space in order to collate observations of their own children. This 'developmental psychology' was elucidated by Gessel at Yale in 1911.

In the 1920s, Gessel's 'Psycho-clinic' incorporated a small, well-lit laboratory sided by two-way mirrors. The experimenter and child could not see the observers and camera technician as the scientist (in white coat) was observed 'testing' the child.[4] Rose states:

'The child is here caught up within a complicated
arrangement that will transform it into a...
analysable object, within a particular rational
scientific discourse (developmental psychology)
making a particular kind of claim upon our attention

– a claim to truth.'5

For critics this is psy at its most naïve: practitioners and experimenters act as if the experimental and observational context is irrelevant to the behaviour observed.

The roots of populist psy have more to do with control than liberation, control that for Foucault and Rose is now vested in governmentality via the discourse of individual 'responsibility'. Pilgrim and Treacher summarize in relation to psy therapeutics: 'Psychological therapies, counselling and health education are examples, par excellence, of a new type of moral regulation favoured by government and public.'6

Electricity has been harnessed as an aspect of governmentality. Gessel was an early exponent of a continuing chain of experimentation recorded on film, tape, digital cameras, cell-phone, You-tube, etc. For citizens going about their everyday business, the clocking-in machines of factories have been replaced by technological monitoring of modern office entrances, police officers walking the beat in town centres are supplanted by CCTV, the 'Eye-in-the-Sky' of satellites is sold to us as all-seeing through its privacy-invading portrayal in modern spy movies and the lap-top that demands particular use of keys renders obsolete user-controlled alternatives like pen and ink.

Through the use of cameras prisons and psychiatric wards are no longer only metaphorical panoptica and, for the bad and mad, the electric chair, electrotorture and electroshock, 'pertain to electrocution as a 'clean' technique of bodily coercion.'[7]

Such 'bodily coercion' is maintained by the estimated 10,000 mental health apps now available (see Normality and Novels). 'Mental' activity cannot be monitored. Instead, citizens self-monitor events supposedly related to 'mental health' – sleep patterns, 'positive' and 'negative' thoughts (the categories defined according to social desirability), exercise, etc.

Electricity and its effects are frequently invisible. We might observe CCTV cameras but we don't know if they are switched on. Nonetheless panoptical impact is unaltered. For Anat Pick it 'exudes ambivalent powers: visible and imperceptible, life giving and lethal, healing and punitive.'[8]

For Esther Greenwood, narrator and main character of Sylvia Plath's *The Bell Jar*, the threat of forthcoming electroshock governs through fear. In the opening paragraph, she explicitly compares it to the electrocution of the Rosenbergs and later describes her first shock treatment in much the same way:

'Then something bent down and took hold of me and shook me like the end of the world. Whee-ee-ee-ee-ee, it shrilled, through an air crackling with blue light, and with each flash a great jolt drubbed me till I thought my bones would break and the sap fly out of me like a split plant. I wondered what terrible thing it was I had done.'[9]

Psy practitioners and their institutions are linked via networks of professions, praxis and governmentality to such an extent that the majority will be – often unconsciously – linked to wounding events (see Death-making and David Reville). Wounding practice starts when a person is 'marked' (labelled in ways not valued by the wider society and thus more likely to be confused with others with similar, frequently poorly defined and stigmatizing, labels). This inscription of the self is integral to psy praxis – research, assessment, therapeutics and publication (see Inscription and Insulin coma).

Without some form of inscription, modern discourse could not function. The particular form dominating psy – diagnosis is, however, frequently the beginning of physical and psychological treatments that harm persons. The process of psy assessment and form of discourse taken form part of the gaze and, hence, governmentality.

Psy professions (whose practitioners are also governed in the ways described above) function within more explicit forms of governmentality via electronic record keeping, cameras in institutional spaces, name badges and codes of conduct from professional bodies. Like prison panoptica these forms of the gaze are maintained by those in authority. As with the unseen footage of CCTV cameras on the street, however, only an assumption of the gaze is necessary.

Thus, electronic records are randomly rather than continuously audited, name badges can only be enforced if they allow access (sometimes digital) to places of work and only marginal aspects of codes of conduct (for example, the precise nature of entries to the electronic record) can be strictly enforced. Individual practitioners remain in the position that one-to-one patient contact is rarely observed by others. Patients are not protected by a professional's code of conduct. They are protected by the inward gaze of the professional, an essentially moral discourse.

This can be a precarious position. The history of psychiatry and psychology is replete with examples of abusive practitioners. Electroshock provides an ideal method for both consciously and unconsciously (see Sadism and Spike Milligan) harming people. Porter Phillips noted that shock therapy (via cardiazol) so terrified patients, it rendered them more compliant to other approaches and brought about an alteration in attitude, ' ... so that nursing control and management is carried out with greater ease.'[10]

Images of *One Flew Over the Cuckoo's Nest* remain in the public eye. For all its marketing of electroshock as 'safe and effective' and the promotion of the technology as 'improved' ordinary people are likely to be sceptical of the benefits of applying electric shocks to the brain. Death-making and David Reville, History and Hemingway, and Torture in this volume all discuss why that scepticism is merited. As an 'ultimate' rather than preferred treatment, however, electroshock can be seen as an end-point in the system of governmentality applied to unruly and awkward people.

Gene Tierney

Gene Tierney started an affair with Jack Kennedy when she met him while filming *Dragonwyck*.

Briefly reconciled with her husband, she had a second daughter. She divorced in 1952 and was lover to, amongst others, Spencer Tracy, Clark Gable and Tyrone Power. Off-screen during the making of *The Left Hand of God* in 1955, she became hesitant and would begin sobbing with no provocation. She didn't recognize old friends, forgot conversations as soon as they ended and was convinced people were staring at her cross-eyed.

Tierney voluntarily entered a New York City sanatorium and was electroshocked. Incarcerated a second time in Connecticut, she received more. Tierney described the session as 'degrading.' Sylvia Plath's narrator, Esther, makes the point that facing electroshock when knowing its impact can still be an act of defiance; a subversion of governmentality: 'I would have gone down that hall ... with dignity, like a person coolly resigned to execution.'[11]

History and Hemingway

Since attempts to translate the Torah and, later, the Bible from Aramaic and Hebrew to English via Latin, historiographers have been plagued by the dual difficulty of rendering what early non-English writers intended and the contextual problem that words are used differently at different times. Histories of psychiatry present the same difficulty.

For example, historians struggle to understand whether earlier use of words such as depression can be understood in the way the modern term is used. In 1725 Blakemore writes of 'being depressed into deep Sadness and Melancholy', while in 1801 David Daniel Davis's translation of Pinel's *Treatise on Insanity*, rendered *l'abbattement* as 'depression of spirits.' Some readings of historical texts can be almost diametrically opposed. The following brief history should be read with this in mind.

As noted in the introduction, the ancient Egyptians used electric marine rays to treat epilepsy, and the ancient Romans used the current generated by electric rays for the treatment of headaches, gout, and to assist in obstetrical procedures. The journal *Electricity and Medicine* was first published in 1744. It was claimed here that electric stimuli could be curative for 'neurologic and mental cases of paralysis and epilepsy'.[1]

In 1752 Benjamin Franklin, who sustained two electric shocks himself inflicting minor retrograde amnesia, recorded the use of an 'electro static machine to cure a woman of hysterical fits'.[2] In the 1755 edition of *Electricity and Medicine*, J. B. LeRoy detailed a case of hysterical blindness cured with three applications of electric shock. In 1787, John Birch, an English physician used electric shocks trying to help a popular and suicidal singer.

In 1849, English psychiatrist Charles Bucknill used electrical stimulation of the skin and potassium oxide with melancholic asylum patients. By then Duchenne, the 'father of electrotherapy', was to say: 'No sincere neurologist could practise without the use of electrotherapy.'[3]

George Beard's promotion of the term 'neurasthenia' led Erb, a German neurologist, via a form of inverted deductive reasoning, to conclude that stimulation of the nervous system would cure the disordered nerves. He pioneered electrotherapy. In the USA, Beard went on to co-author a volume of eventually some 600 pages entitled *Medical and Surgical Uses of Electricity*.[4] Beard's treatment (electrical stimulation, rest cure and friendly moral exhortation) was entirely in keeping with his theory that symptoms were, essentially, a result of exhaustion brought on by excessive 'brain work' in bourgeois patients.

These individuals suffered depletion in their bodily energies that were a natural part of human efforts to work and achieve – an optimistic view of humanity Cushman notes as 'very American'.[5] Similar experiments were continuing at the Bicêtre in Paris.[6]

In an 1884 article on the benefits of electricity, Neuth writes:

> 'The therapeutic value of electricity in mental disease is not by any means hypothetical only ... So long ago as 1804 Galvani's nephew, Aldini is reported as having cured two cases of melancholia by galvanism ... prior to this we read that Dr Bischoff of Jena and Dr Augustin of Berlin cured several cases of insanity with paralysis by galvanism.'[7]

He says of a suicidal woman inscribed as melancholic at the Sussex Asylum: 'Electricity was applied 26 times, positive pole to head, negative to hand. At first, she could only bear a very few cells, six or eight, and it seemed to make her head ache – however, she was afterwards able to bear more.'

He added that the results were 'very satisfactory', saying that she was 'much brighter, converses rationally' and 'has no desire for self-destruction'.[8]

Patients might be given a shock from a Leyden jar (a device for storing electric charge) or, after being insulated, the patient would be electrified and sparks drawn from the affected part. Apart from these examples, there are more forerunners to electroshock involving actual electricity (rather than eels or camphor) than might be supposed. For example, at Ticehurst Asylum in 1901 one patient was given '...the electrical battery for his cataleptic trance.' And another, the electric battery applied to his head and neck for, '...slow cerebration.'[9]

Electric shock updated the pre-occupation that medicine had with establishing physical cures for life's ills. Trepanning, for example, far from disappearing with the ancient Egyptians, re-emerged with Roger of Salerno in the twelfth century and again in 1899 with Claye Shaw at Banstead Asylum. Rather than freeing spirits, Shaw was attempting to relieve inter-cranial pressure, a presumed cause of general paresis.[10] The site of inter-cranial pressure was the brain, an organ so little known and so complex that psychiatry has not hesitated to claim jurisdiction over its workings and modification.

In the early part of twentieth century, neurologists vied with neurosurgeons and psychiatrists for dominance in the field. The first group saw neurosurgeons as useful partners in the enterprise. Psychiatrists were regarded as a profession that should limit themselves to functional disorders of conduct and an ill-defined 'mind'. For psychiatry, however, the brain seemed to show some promise in demonstrating that functional disorders were physically based.[11]

In the 1930s, a Hungarian psychiatrist, Julius Nyirö, promoted a theory that schizophrenia could not coexist with epilepsy. Ergo, if epilepsy could be induced in someone diagnosed with schizophrenia, the schizophrenia would be cured. László Meduna claimed dramatic success with a catatonic schizophrenic after injecting camphor (used as a stimulant for centuries in China and Japan) to induce convulsions. Meduna instigated shock treatment using the synthetic metrazol.[12] Bini and Cerletti, two Italian psychiatrists, are credited with the move from chemically to electrically induced convulsions. They first diagnosed and then electrocuted a vagrant and declared him 'cured'. He agreed. In similar vein, at a Shropshire seminar over 60 years later, Viv Lindow, a shock survivor and researcher, explained to a group of psychiatrists that the way to avoid further shocks and get out of psychiatric hospital is to say you feel better, however you feel.[13]

Accounts of Bini's first foray into electroshock differ in terms of emphasis and translation. Two of the most thorough accounts take subtly different positions. Edward Shorter and Eliot Valenstein agree on the date – though Shorter is more specific; April 18 1938 as opposed to Valenstein's 'April.' As is well known, Bini and Cerletti (with the assistance of Ferdinando Accornero and two others) had set up a primitive electroshock device on the second floor of the Clinic for Nervous and Mental Diseases at the University of Rome where Cerletti had been chief since 1935.

On April 15, the police had referred a 39 year-old engineer from Milan who had been found wandering about the railroad station. Inscribed as schizophrenic, the man was electroshocked through both temples with first 80, then 90 and finally 100 volts. For Valenstein, between the second and third shock, the victim says, 'Not another one! It's deadly!'[14]

Minor variants of this reading have been repeated in a number of volumes on electroshock. Shorter's account renders a more refined translation: 'Look out! The first is pestiferous, the second mortiferous.'[15] Both versions agree that after the third convulsion and forty eight seconds of unconsciousness the man responds in answer to the question 'What happened to you?': 'I don't know. Maybe I was asleep.'

Shorter goes on to say that, after a further eleven electroshocks, the patient, 'did, in fact, get well.'[16] For Valenstein, the story ends with the third shock.

Ernest Hemingway

By late 1960, despite his literary success, Ernest Hemingway was constantly worried about money and his safety. He worried about taxes and that he would never return to Cuba to retrieve manuscripts left in a bank vault. He believed the FBI was actively monitoring his movements at his home in Ketchum, Idaho. The FBI had, in fact, opened a file on him during World War II, when he used his boat the *Pilar* to patrol the waters off Cuba.

J. Edgar Hoover had an agent in Havana watching Hemingway during the 1950s. By the end of November, 1960, his friend and physician George Saviers suggested Hemingway go to the Mayo Clinic in Minnesota. In an attempt to maintain anonymity, he was checked in under Saviers' name, but the FBI knew he was at the Clinic (later documented in a letter written by an agent in January 1961). He was given electroshock as many as 15 times in December 1960 and was 'released in ruins' in January 1961.

Visited by his friend Aaron Hotchner, editor,

biographer, novelist and playwright,[17] Hemingway said:

> 'Well, what is the sense of ruining my head and erasing my memory, which is my capital, and putting me out of business? It was a brilliant cure but we lost the patient.'[18]

Ironically, it may well have been the combination of medications given to Hemingway that created the so called depressive state for which he was treated.

One morning, three months after his release from the Mayo Clinic, Hemingway's wife Mary found him holding a shotgun in the kitchen in their Ketchum home. She called Saviers, who sedated him and admitted him to the Sun Valley Hospital; from there he was returned to the Mayo Clinic for more electroshock. He was released in late June and arrived home on June 30.

Two days later, in the early morning hours of July 2 1961, in his entrance foyer Ernest Hemingway shot himself with his favourite shotgun.

Inscription
and Insulin coma

In this volume the term inscription is preferred to diagnosis or labelling in relation to the Psy complex.[1] Medical, clinical and therapeutic notes 'fix' the recipient of psychiatric and psychological services using a particular, frequently technical, language at a certain time and place.

Once inscribed, the continuation of notes or an electronic record makes it likely that future professionals will use that inscription as a reference point for further examination and intervention. In medical settings this may be essential to a person's care – it is important for a surgeon, say, to know that a cancer has been located in a person's liver and the word carcinoma will lead to particular surgical and other medical interventions.

Confusion results, however, from the nature of the arcane lexicon of psy. For example, schizophrenia, schizotypal and schizoid all have distinct definitions (if not construct validity), but the prefix 'schiz' is likely to lead to similarly labelled people being treated as if they all required the same intervention.

In the case of electroshock, this is particularly true for the term 'depression' where a range of potentially helpful and humane interventions are replaced by electrocution of the inscribed person.

Psychological and psychiatric praxis focuses on character and conduct, frequently framing that conduct as 'disease.' Psychiatric diagnoses, however, have neither construct validity nor reliability (see Evidence and Electrocution). The inscription of certain 'problems', for example, exhaustion due to overwork (diagnosed as depression) is privileged over less socially acceptable aspects of the person's character, such as preferring work to family life.

A person's conduct will be marked as exceptional and deserving of a psy inscription if the professional sees elements of, say, checking as extreme and therefore 'obsessional', or quietude as 'withdrawn' and thus 'depressed'. Similarly a teacher might ask for an assessment of possible Attention Deficit Hyperactivity Disorder (ADHD) if his or her attention is repeatedly drawn to a particular child rather than the others in the classroom. Inscription as an aspect of governmentality (see Governmentality and Gene Tierney), helps construct the social order and disqualifies challenges to it.

Inscriptions of the self posthumously continue; we are remembered or celebrated in obituaries with the same descriptors we have accrued throughout life. Colleagues, family and friends may continue to use these individualized descriptors (brave, weak, foolish, a 'good' father or 'intelligent' person, etc.) long after our physical death. For those inscribed by psy professionals, their mark as a 'schizophrenic' may long outlive descriptors such as 'dad', 'electrician' or 'sister'. Obituaries consistently privilege the eye-catching over the mundane and the same is true for bereaved relatives who may refer to the dead person in terms of his or her 'suffering' from 'mental illness.' Terms such as 'depressed' and 'autistic' are now part of the vernacular. An official inscription tends to cast them in stone. For a child of an inscribed parent genetic hypotheses concerning distress make it likely that parental inscriptions will be the starting point of any investigation by a psy professional with access to the parent's patient record. The opportunity to listen to the child's explanations for what might be wrong in the child's life is lost as professionals assume problems lie within the child's genetic make-up.

Official inscriptions of the self can be based on the slightest of evidence. In the famous Kinsey Report purporting to delineate the sexual habits of the average American citizen, for example, discussion of the sexual behaviour of 317 boys 'was in fact culled from the diaries of one paedophile'.[2]

Psy inscribes and disciplines the self through language and direct intervention. The language of technopraxis pervades modernist discourse, promoting inscription of the public self. Within professional discourse a lack of reflexivity results in theories, research and psy interventions founded in language that consistently has no parameters beyond itself. Psy professionals are involved in a social rather than scientific process where an unexamined lexicon of 'disorder', 'progress' and so on is accepted as part of a broader psy project.

That lexicon can be found daily in the media.

Journalists can be accurate, neutral (editors can change things) and occasionally crass. The UK's *Daily Telegraph* includes examples of all three forms of writing in between half page photographs of everything from birds catching struggling fish to Royal family engagements and adverts. The rugby pages from the 22 December 2017 deserve a special mention. The article is humdrum, but the headline 'Northampton require some shock therapy' is on the dark side. Perhaps the writer didn't know just how many of his older readers had already been there, done that.[3]

Similarly, in an otherwise gripping account of recent British politics Andrew Marr casually describes the media pre-occupation with the 'sixties as having an, 'almost autistic repetitiveness...'[4] Inscribing an entire industry does have the advantage that everyone is equal. This mirrors Spitzer and his colleagues' intention when revising the *Diagnostic and Statistical Manual* (*DSM-III*) in 1980 that anyone could be caught in the diagnostic net. *Time* magazine reported from the first of their meetings that the most important thing, 'is that DSM-III is of crucial importance to the profession [because] ... its diagnoses are generally recognized by the courts, hospitals and insurance companies.'[5] The American Psychiatric Association (APA) committee continues to *vote* new psychiatric disorders into the *DSM*.

One of the first published accounts of madness – largely using the words of the patient and written in 1810 – was produced by John Haslam, apothecary (resident medical officer) to Bethlem Hospital, London, during its move from Moorfields to Lambeth.[6] Like his contemporaries, Haslam saw reason and insanity as opposites; 'comprehensive taxonomies of madness were quite worthless. Insanity was better seen as a single basic disorder, visible in a variety of phases and manifestations.'[7] Madness was 'the opposite to reason and good sense, as light is to darkness, straight to crooked, &c'.[8]

It wasn't until the 1830s that books about insanity came to regularly include clinical vignettes and reports of subjective experience: so-called 'elementary' symptoms.[9] There was a marked difference over a period of barely 50 years between the work of Haslam, Rush and Pinel and that of Esquirol, Morel and Tuke. There were few diagnostic groupings prior to the 1830s; melancholia, mania, phrenitis, delirium, paranoia, lethargy, carus and dementia were the main ones.

As new nosologies appeared, so did new categories; others, such as carus and phrenitis, all but disappeared. In Germany, first Krafft-Ebing in 1867 and then Westphal used a technical term – *Zwangsvorstellung* – to refer to irresistible thoughts (obsessions in contemporary discourse). In France, Falret in 1866 had already used the term 'obsession' and Morel had written about emotion as a foundation to the onset of obsessionality. Later, Luys brought subjective experience to the fore by defining obsessions as private, individual events.

By the end of the century, Esquirol, Ball, Magnan, Kahlbaum, Kraepelin and Maudsley were some of the more renowned nosologists to have produced extensive and competing classifications of psychiatric morbidity. In 1906, the Joint College of the Royal College of Physicians of London drew up the fourth edition of the *Nomenclature of Diseases*, forerunner to the *International Classification of Diseases*, now in its eleventh edition. The publication of yet another classificatory scheme was not universally welcomed; in his presidential address to the American Medico-Psychological Association, Charles Hill the following year observed the only diagnosis omitted was 'the classifying mania of medical authors'.[10]

The first *Statistical Manual for the Use of Institutions for the Insane* was published in 1918. Mental disorders were now divided into two main categories: disturbance resulting from impairment of brain function (trauma, alcoholism, multiple sclerosis, etc.) and disorders resulting from an inability to adjust. The second group was further divided into psychotic and psychoneurotic disorders.

Between 1948 and its publication in 1952, the APA Committee on Nomenclature and Statistics circulated for comment a draft *Diagnostic and Statistical Manual* (*DSM-I*) to numerous organisations and individuals. Post-war, the psychiatric community, influenced by psychodynamic theory, moved towards a position whereby mental health and illness were on a continuum and sought to treat more individuals diagnosed as psychoneurotic. *DSM-II* was published in 1968.

Its authors turned their sights to the wider community for corroboration and collaboration. Influenced by the eighth edition of the *International*

Classification of Diseases (ICD-8), affective reactions became major affective disorders, now including involutional melancholia and listing psychotic depressive reaction separately. The overall number of disorders rose to 163. *DSM-III*, published in 1980, contained 265 potential inscriptions.

A new feature of *DSM-III* was its multiaxial orientation, Axis I describing symptom-based disorders, Axis II personality disorders. The remaining three axes specified medical conditions (an intriguing feature in a nosology supposedly articulating all psychiatric inscriptions as medical phenomena), severity of stressors and the best level of psychological functioning during the preceding year. The all-encompassing nature of the new volume was commented on by Jay Katz, a professor of psychiatry at Yale: 'If you look at *DSM-III* you can classify all of us under one rubric or another of mental disorder.'[11]

Freud, Marie Jahoda and Karl Menninger were amongst many psy professionals to already be on record as suggesting that we are all mentally ill at one time or another, to a greater or lesser degree. This position puts those frequently critical of the diagnostic endeavour, for example, clinical psychologists, in a paradoxical position from which they can escape via the Judeo-Christian tradition of charitableness.

Distress can be normalised or placed on a continuum wherein it is the suffering of the individual or others (for example, the family) or the temporary apparent inability to function socially (so-called 'problems in living') that dictate the need for professional intervention; suffering is the only justification needed for referral to a mental health professional.

DSM-III-R, DSM-IV and *DSM-IV-TR* were published in 1987, 1994 and 2000 respectively. The 265 diagnoses in *DSM-III* increased to 292 for *DSM-III-R* and 365 for both the later editions. *DSM-5*, published in 2013, has a similar total.

Like the use of psychiatric medications, electroshock use is, in any case, neither consistent nor inscription-specific across the world. It is forbidden in Slovenia (whatever the diagnosis) though a small number of patients are referred outside to Zagreb, Croatia where the procedure is still used. Slovenian authorities claim only 3 to 12 patients are referred each year.

In Greece, a 2007 survey found 137 people were given electroshock (Greece has a population of about 11.3 million), a rate of 0.001 per cent of the population. Schizophrenia was the most common diagnosis. In Turkey one hospital (Bakirkoy Research and Training Hospital for Psychiatric and Neurological Diseases in Istanbul) accounted for 3,490 electroshock recipients from 2008–2010, the majority with a diagnosis of mania or schizophrenia.[12]

Such disparate usage reflects the origins of electroshock. Variants had been used with people inscribed with catalepsy, hysteria, melancholia and epilepsy for over a hundred and fifty years though it wasn't until the 1940s that Western psychiatry narrowed its focus (see History and Hemingway).

Now the focus is expanding again with zealous

psychiatrists prescribing electroshock for children inscribed as autistic and bi-polar.

The route to ending inscription by psy – if not the general public – is easier than the above might suppose. Robbie Piper, a primary school teacher in the north of England has noted that formal diagnosis of ADHD has fallen off in the last year as his local authority has been unable to fill their two educational psychologist posts.[13] The less inscribers, the fewer inscriptions.

Insulin coma

Insulin coma therapy involved injecting people with insulin in order to induce coma. It was first attempted for people inscribed with schizophrenia at the Lichterfeld Hospital in Berlin by Manfred Sakel in 1927, then later in Vienna.[14] He suggested that the rationale was to 'overstimulate the vagus system', adding that psychotherapy might continue as part of the treatment.[15]

Joseph Wortis, psychiatrist and eventually founding editor of the journal *Biological Psychiatry* observed Sakel practicing insulin coma in 1935 and introduced it to the USA. In 1936, on the invitation of Frederick Pearson, State Commissioner of Mental Hygiene, Sakel emigrated to New York. Once there he widely promoted insulin shock (see Zealotry and Zelda Fitzgerald). He reported an initial recovery rate of 87 per cent, to be amended to 12–14 per cent in the USA by 1939.[16]

Despite that revision to outcome success, by the late 1940s the majority of psychiatric hospitals in the US were using it. UK psychiatrists from the Board of

Control visited Vienna in 1935 and 1936, and within two years 31 hospitals in England and Wales also had insulin treatment units. In his account of directing the 'insulin room' at Warlingham Park Hospital in Surrey, England, between 1948 and 1953, Ronald Sandison discusses the outcome of insulin therapy for two patients undergoing 45 and 52 induced comas in a context where 'no one said: 'This is what you should be doing, this is where you should look.'[17] The experimental nature of the treatment seemed of little concern to the author, a Jungian analyst by inclination (see Research and Robeson).

Insulin coma was labour-intensive and required trained staff and a special unit. Patients, usually inscribed with schizophrenia, were selected on the basis of having a good prognosis and the physical strength to withstand an arduous treatment (with no standard guidelines). Typically, injections were administered six days a week for about two months.

The daily insulin dose was gradually increased to 100–150 units until comas were produced, at which point the dose would be levelled out. Occasionally doses of up to 450 units were used. After 50 or 60 comas, or earlier if the psychiatrist thought that maximum benefit had been achieved, the dose of insulin was rapidly reduced before treatment was stopped. Courses of up to two years were not unknown.

After the injection patients would experience various symptoms of decreased blood glucose: flushing, pallor, perspiration, salivation, drowsiness or restlessness. Sopor and coma – if the dose was high enough – would follow. Each coma would last for up to an hour and be terminated by intravenous glucose or via a naso-gastric tube. Seizures sometimes occurred before or during the coma. Many patients would be tossing, rolling, moaning, twitching, having spasms or thrashing around.

Many psychiatrists regarded seizures as therapeutic and patients were sometimes electroshocked or given cardiazol/metrazol convulsive therapy during the coma, or on the day of the week when they didn't have insulin treatment (see History and Hemingway). When they were not in a coma, insulin coma patients were kept together in a group and given special treatment and attention. The most severe risks of insulin coma therapy were death and brain damage, resulting from irreversible or prolonged coma respectively. Estimates of risk of death range from one to five per cent of recipients.

Psychiatric nurses were instructed to take their insulin patients out walking and occupy them with games and competitions, flower-picking, map-reading, etc. Patients actually required continuous supervision as there was a danger of hypoglycaemic aftershocks after the coma.[18]

In a 1953 article, Bourne argued that there was no sound basis for believing that insulin coma therapy counteracted the schizophrenic process in a specific way. If treatment worked, he said, it was because patients were chosen for their good prognosis and were given special treatment: 'insulin patients tend to be an elite group sharing common privileges and perils'.[19]

As use of electroshock increased in the 1950s, insulin coma was less used. For example, in 1956 in Severalls Hospital, Essex, UK, insulin coma was given to 39 patients, 18 patients received modified insulin coma and 432 patients were electroshocked.[20]

Although insulin treatment was on the wane in the USA, Mayer-Gross and colleagues could write, in 1960, that it 'is still recognised as one of the most effective methods of treating early schizophrenia'.[21] It was unmentioned in psychiatric textbooks within ten years and does not appear at all in the index of Stone's history of psychiatric treatment, *Healing the Mind*.[22]

For many people the change came too late. Leonard Roy Frank, a US-based activist, says of his experience of the procedure: 'I was forced to undergo combined insulin-electroshock, a total of 85 shock 'treatments'... My father had signed the consent form.'[23] Walter Freeman (see Zealotry and Zelda Fitzgerald) might have argued that Frank's recovery and spirited fight against psychiatry over some 50 years was evidence that electroshock had not harmed him, despite Frank's assertions to the contrary and the fact he lost his memory for the two years preceding the first shock.

Justification
and Janet Frame

Just as the theories of Hegar and of Shallmayer became part of the justificatory rhetoric for forced sterilization in the early years of the twentieth century, similar theories led to explicit or implicit (via 'mercy based' euthanasia) genocide over the next thirty years.

In the late 1930s the theory of degeneration with its blend of biology and implications for state welfare and economic health justified death-making in psychiatric hospitals in Germany (see Death-making and David Reville). Justificatory rhetoric is rife in all branches of medicine often distilled into 'doctor knows best.' Typically, electroshock is justified as a 'life-saver' (see Marketing and Movies) or, in the case of older recipients, 'better' than potentially dangerous drugs.

Rhetoric demands that the speaker uses tropes familiar to the listener to support a position. Tropes such as 'science' or 'research' are aimed at allaying recipient fears about harm and adverse effects. Expert authority is granted to the psy professional who must persuade the recipient using a combination of supposed data to which the patient doesn't have access and key phrases such as 'safe and effective.'

Additionally, there are tales of psychiatrists who add to their persuasiveness via appeals to a form of referent power – they say that if they were depressed, they would willingly be electroshocked.[1] Such statements are not, necessarily, without foundation; there are, for example, accounts of the consultant psychiatrists at Shelton Hospital, Shropshire in the late 1950s electroshocking *each other*.

In December 2017, the *Daily Telegraph* reported a UK NHS survey suggesting that a 'growing reliance' by the public on anti-depressants had fuelled a 47 per cent rise in prescription drugs over the previous ten years. The survey of over 8,000 adults showed that a quarter were on at least three drugs while 'millions of pensioners are on at least five types of medication.' The 47 percent rise involved over a million prescriptions; one in ten English adults are estimated to be on anti-depressants, a six per cent rise in two years. The highest level of prescription was for women between the ages of 16 and 24.

Helen Stokes-Lampard, from the Royal College of General Practitioners, justifies the rise in prescription for anti-depressants by suggesting that people are, 'more likely to seek help.' Prescriptions for blood pressure tablets medications and statins top the list.[2] No mention is made of the financial incentives for GPs to prescribe these drugs nor the pharma and psy-backed promotion of the idea of depression; inscription of depression and anxiety has risen 20 per cent in five years.

The rate of obesity is now claimed to be 50 per cent. No link is made between the rise in anti-depressant use and its impact on exercise and appetite.

The report may be read as offering many examples

of self-interest; profits for drug companies, inscriptions that lead to state benefits and the way in which conduct inscribed as illness loses its moral dimension leading to personal agency being removed for people who might otherwise be described as sad or lazy. Instead, people are inscribed as 'suffering' from 'depression' – the zeitgeist of a no-blame culture renders alternative explanations 'insensitive'.

As a libertarian Szasz did not hesitate to describe people seeking inscription and prescription as indolent, work-shy or bad rather than mad. 'Help-seeking' behaviour must be justified in terms of inability or incapacity. Thus, people can claim they are 'too depressed' to get out of bed, look after the kids, go to work, enjoy relationships, and so on. Criminal conduct can be justified with a similar appeal to an internal (and, thus invisible) uncontrollable urge.

The voice of G-d spoke clearly to the prophets. For those who claim that same voice insists they cut themselves, attack a shop-keeper or wander naked through a park there are psy professionals who can justify the urge by reference to theories of bio-chemical imbalance, historic child-abuse and so on.

Stokes-Lampard justifies the increased patient visits to GPs by reference to the patients' motivation. She does not see a reason to justify GPs' willingness to agree to those same appointments and prescriptions; her sub-text might be that GPs are the passive recipients of the misery of others.

Some conduct and many systems require little justification. If we value life, it makes sense to drive under speed limits imposed because slower speeds are safer amongst other drivers observing the same restrictions. If we regard some criminals as dangerous or likely to re-offend and we want to give society a break from their actions, then prison makes sense.

Both examples, however, lie within a moralizing discourse; protection of others through safer driving or people and property through incarceration of offenders are both seen as being for the greater good. Opinions differ on what the greater good might be; Psy interventions are a form of moral orthopaedics.[3]

Bruce Levine lists ten conscious and unconscious ways in which psy professionals do harm. His tenth is: Hypocrisy over conflict of interest: 'Professionals have great power to 'maintain their cash flow.' They can, for example, sell patients the idea that episodic depression is a chemical-imbalance disease like diabetes, and that they need to be on medication for life. They can sabotage patients' other relationships by focusing on – and helping exaggerate – minor frustrations with friends or intimates, resulting in patients becoming isolated and dependent on the professional.

The professional's job ceases when treatment is successful, and so professionals who are doing their job well are working against themselves financially ... Also, patients not only have severe long-term adverse effects from psychiatric medications but from electroconvulsive therapy (ECT).'[4]

This kind of analysis is likely to be rejected by members of psy who prefer to be seen as caring, self-less, scientific or acting 'professionally'. Their own self-justifying rhetoric need only be based on the Judeo-Christian notion of 'charitableness' – actions are justified as beneficently responding to suffering. For patients, a denial of this position and a refutation of the physician's care and expertise can be isolating. The patient still feels in need of succour but is set adrift by cynicism.

Electroshock survivors can find some support in the many patient and survivor groups to be found locally or on the Internet. But if they also deny that essential component of psy justification – an inscription – they will no longer receive state benefits or the internalised excuse of 'illness.' Szasz's version of libertarianism can be bleak; echoing Sartre, we are not responsible for the cards we are dealt, but we are responsible for playing them.

The justification for electroshock relies on several rhetorical moves. Most of us are familiar with health/illness and responsible/non-responsible dichotomies. Within such a discourse the notions of cause and effect and progression are paramount. A person advised that a cut might lead to an infection and ultimately gangrene is likely to clean the cut before infection can take hold and, if that fails, to apply antibiotic cream. To not do so would be seen as irresponsible. Many people are cautious about cuts for themselves and their children.

For psy, issues of cause and effect, progression and responsibility are conflated within an illusory dichotomy of health/illness, a dichotomy eroded by concepts such as 'spectrum'. People are inscribed with fictional illnesses (depression, schizophrenia, etc.), informed that such illness may progress (from, say, ADHD to ADD) and that they are responsible for ameliorating their 'disorder' via accepting moral orthopaedics, medication or electroshock.

There is no evidence that so-called psy conditions progress (although medication may well make matters worse) and, for those treated involuntarily, 'responsibility' is a moveable feast; people are seen as responsible for complying with medical instruction but not sufficiently responsible to live their lives as they see fit (see Law and Lou Reed).

The libertarian and institutional psy positions revolve around an inherently conflictual view of choice. For Szasz, a homeless indigent person who acts in ways likely to lead to inscription and incarceration is choosing to act in these ways and is being rewarded by the state or guilty parents by the provision of somewhere to live. If people commit criminal offences they can be rewarded by being spared prison in favour of psychiatric treatment or incarceration.[5]

The role of psy here is to support the person's (false) claim to a lack of choice due to an inscribable 'disorder'. For professionals abjuring a disorder discourse, the person's defence can be that the behaviour could not be otherwise because of historic factors in the person's past – for example, someone who has lashed out in a public place may have done so because he or she was 'overwhelmed' by memories of assault as a child. The choice to lash out is lost within such an explanation. A custodial sentence may be avoided if the psy professional offers a form of psychic archaeology to 'bring closure' to the past memories.

Beyond the criminal justice system, professional justifications of another's behaviour that assume a lack of choice thrive in a context where professional justifications for treatment regimens take precedent. In the case of electroshock, justificatory rhetoric around the shock itself has been forced to shift from convulsion to charge. The suggestion of potential progression might be used to 'nip the condition' in the bud because of signs of 'suicidality' (see Evidence and Electrocution). Appeals to the mysteries of brain bio-chemistry and neuronal firing may be referred to in recommending 'maintenance' electroshock (see Opposition and Oprah Winfrey and Kindness and Kitty Dukakis).

For Szasz, this is a charade. People are pretending they don't choose to behave in asocial ways or can't face difficult events and join in a kind of *folie à deux* with professionals who go along with them for the sake of earning money as experts. For Peter Breggin, patients are refusing to face how tough life is and turn to psy as a crutch, albeit one that can end up destroying brain cells.[6]

Community and socially aware psychologists and psychiatrists might take issue with such accounts based on privileging a discourse of individualism. Explanations of conduct might be seen through the prisms of poverty and power (although, in the case of electroshock in the USA, it is actually the better off who are recipients due to its cost). This form of justificatory rhetoric may not be shared by service recipients, but has the advantage that electroshock is no answer to poverty.

It may, however, answer the profit motive. An APA survey found that 72 per cent of electroshocks were paid for by insurance companies.[7] One psychiatrist had previously commented: 'Finding that the patient had insurance seemed like the most common indication of giving electroshock.'[8]

Over twenty-five years ago, Frank calculated that in the USA electroshock had become a $2-3 billion-a-year industry suggesting that, with the overall cost for a series of shocks in a private hospital ranging from $10,000 to $25,000 shock doctors could earn an additional $200,000 per annum.[9] A moderate rate of inflation suggests a potential additional $300,000 annual income as one justification for electroshock.

Janet Frame (Birth name: Nene Janet PatersoClutha, 1924-2004)

In September 1945, the New Zealand author Janet Frame left her teacher-training classroom at Dunedin's Arthur Street School during a visit from an inspector. She was briefly admitted to the psychiatric ward of the local Dunedin hospital for observation.

Frame was unwilling to return home to her family, frequently a place of anger and violence between her brother and father. She was transferred from the local hospital's psychiatric ward to Seacliff Lunatic Asylum, 20 miles north of Dunedin. Over the following eight years, Frame was repeatedly readmitted, usually voluntarily, to psychiatric hospitals in addition to Seacliff; these included Avondale Lunatic Asylum, in Auckland, and Sunnyside Hospital in Christchurch. First inscribed with schizophrenia, she was subjected to electroshock and insulin coma.

In 1951, while Frame was still a patient at Seacliff, New Zealand's Caxton Press published her first book, a collection of short stories (*The Lagoon and Other Stories*). The volume was awarded the Hubert Church Memorial Award, one of New Zealand's most prestigious literary prizes. Her scheduled lobotomy was cancelled.

Frame left New Zealand in late 1956. Over the next seven years she wrote four novels and a volume of short stories. She lived and worked in Europe, primarily based in London as well as Ibiza and Andorra. Feeling overwhelmed she admitted herself to the Maudsley in London, where the psychiatrist Alan Miller said that she had never suffered from schizophrenia.

In an effort to alleviate the ill-effects of her years spent in and out of psychiatric hospitals, she began regular therapy sessions with psychiatrist Robert Cawley, who encouraged her to pursue her writing. Frame dedicated seven of her novels to him.[10]

An Angel at My Table, published in 1984, is the second of Frame's three autobiographies and the title of the 1990 film made by Jane Campion covering Frame's life from childhood to successful author. The first and third volumes are *To the Is-Land* (1982) and *The Envoy from Mirror City* (1984).[8] *An Angel at My Table* was the first film from New Zealand to be screened at the Venice Film Festival, where it was awarded the Grand Special Jury (see Marketing and Movies).

For her final novel, *The Carpathians* (1989), she was awarded the Commonwealth Writers' Prize. In the Queen's Birthday Honours 1983 she was appointed Commander of the Order of the British Empire (CBE) for services to literature. She died in Dunedin in January 2004, aged 79, from acute myeloid leukaemia.

Killing with Kindness
and Kitty Dukakis

I have held three beloved family pet dogs as they died. All three were ill and had been in great pain. As dogs do, they still had an appetite but walks were out of the question. All three were given a sedative before the vet injected them with pentobarbital, a seizure medication. Like the 'execution' of Resi Noth's dog in *Mother Night*, Sam, Ralph and Mara died 'without a shudder.'[1] They lie, wrapped in their blankets slowly joining the earth in Myddlewood, their graves marked and trees growing around them. Their lives had been full, their enjoyment with my children obvious.

Was it a kindness to kill them? Whose suffering had been the greater – their own or that of the family witnessing their increasing disability?

There is an inherent violence in the act of electroshock – to the person, the brain, frequently to the body; as in the case of electroshock without anaesthetic leading to fractures and, potentially to those that witness it. That violence may be carried out in the name of kindness (see Torture for an account of nursing staff roles), an erroneous belief in electroshock as 'life-saving' or with the understanding that violence to the brain and subsequent damage is 'necessary' and a price (to the patient) worth paying.

By far the majority of that violence has been carried

out on the persons and bodies of older women (see Death-making and David Reville and Women). This has been accounted for by reference to the over-representation of female patients in the psy system and justifications concerning the 'danger' of giving older people the only recognized alternative – psychotropic medication.

An unwelcome interpretation is simpler. We live in a gendered and misogynistic society. Globally women are overwhelmed and oppressed by demanding, gendered roles and inequality in financial, physical and other forms of power. Women who get to the top are heralded for equally male-defined characteristics – 'assertiveness' and 'independence' in female politicians, actresses or teenage girls are positioned as both worthy and unusual traits. In more closed systems like the family or an institution, such gendering is less visible but, by definition, these systems reflect and re-inforce the zeitgeist.

What then might a busy, probably tired psychiatrist in a position of power do when confronted by an older female patient who has so far frustrated all efforts by the service to make her improve? One possibility is punishment and, unconsciously or consciously, recourse to the violence of electroshock is punishment. In a fundamentally patriarchal closed system, female as well as male psychiatrists are likely to prescribe electroshock.

There are many examples of psy staff who have been found assaulting and harming patients. Breggin, for example, discusses his early experiences in psychiatric establishments where rape was common.[2] In an essentially closed environment such as a hospital or prison, the ordinary rules of society either don't exist or are not applied. There are cases where psychiatrists have been dismissed for *branding* patients and numerous examples of other abuses of power.

These sometimes come to light and result in public inquiries (see Consent and Clementine Churchill). These inquiries tend to focus on individual maliciousness rather than the inherent abusiveness of clustering unwanted folk in unusual ordered environments that operate as institutional panoptica. In these environments, however, it seems inevitable that a combination of the patriarchal context, internalised demands to be 'caring' and 'scientific' while using mechanistic rather than humane methods as well as simple pressure of work will lead clinicians to seek scapegoats.

Who better than an elderly woman who just won't show signs of 'improvement'? Such an individualistic account would be unpopular with critical psychologists but individualized explanations of the conduct of psy professionals do have the merit of balancing the individualized notions of internal disorder ascribed to patients by those same professionals.

Kindness and concern for the welfare of others may underlie the aspirations of many – hopefully the majority – of psy professionals. When that kindness and concern is rebuffed – either directly by patients or by virtue of a patient's failure to respond to interventions – the professional may react in a resentful or aggressive way. To an extent, the professional's raison d'être is threatened. Some professionals will do some soul searching (if they are of a psycho-analytical bent this will be in the form of an examination of 'counter-transference' in supervision) while others may react by discharging the patient, labelling the person 'treatment-resistant' or referring the patient on.

Bleuler's first use of the term schizophrenia in 1908 had defined the so-called symptoms as inherently incurable – a feature of schizophrenia was that symptom-free individuals were said to be 'in remission' rather than cured. Despite that, Thomas Szasz once remarked that declaring someone inscribed with schizophrenia as 'incurable' was a comment on the skills of the therapist rather than a statement about the patient.[3] The 'treatment resistant' patient is thus one that adds to a professional's sense that either the intervention or the person of the professional is failing.

Either way, referral on is an obvious next step and, as noted in Death-making and David Reville, referral is likely to result in more invasive, potentially harmful, procedures.[4] It is not necessary to invoke *un*-kindness as motivating the referral or the preference among some psychiatrists to use electroshock as the first intervention.

Ordinary discourse would suggest that a professional confronted with failure might wish the patient harm but a sense of duty and care can still result in a harmful, potentially lethal, series of physical interventions for the recipient.

Between 100,000 and 200,000 patients now undergo electroshock in the United States annually. This is only an estimate, however, as only four states (Colorado, California, Texas and Massachusetts) require reporting statistics. The *American Psychiatric Association* claims that one in 200 shock patients suffer memory loss. Figures from California suggest a proportion closer to one in 5. Reporting of adverse effects ('complications') is limited to non-fatal cardiac arrests or arrhythmias requiring resuscitation, fractures, apnoea persisting 20 minutes or more after initiation of treatment, memory loss reported by the patient extending more than three months following the completed course and deaths which occur during or within the first 24 hours after a treatment.

Between 1989 and 1994 (1993 figures were unavailable) over 12,000 people received electroshock, 445 (3.6%) of whom were involuntary patients and 364 (3%) received shock without consent. More than a fifth of all patients had serious complications. The most often reported complication (19.7% of all patients and 93.6% of all complications) was extended memory loss lasting longer than three months.[5]

Between September 1993 and April 1995, the 15,240 shock administrations in Texas hospitals have been subjected to a review. Almost all of the patients (88.1%) were white, five were less than 18 years of age and 70.3 per cent were women. Eight patients died within 14 days of a treatment, three of whom killed themselves. The researchers conclude: 'Our data support the common finding that ECT is generally safe and effective.'[6] At its worst the death rate after electroshock has been estimated at between one and five per cent, usually attributed to adverse reaction to the anaesthesia. Some people are killed with kindness.

Between 1919 and 1933, Henry Cotton had overseen the removal of thousands of teeth, tonsils and parts of the gut and cervix from numerous patients in his search for a cure to the focal infection he was convinced caused psychosis (see Research and Robeson and X-rays). The majority of his patients were women. Despite his (timely?) demise, the last reference to focal infection and surgery was located by Andrew Scull in the Trenton Hospital annual report for 1956. Every year the outstanding member of staff is given the 'Cotton Award for Kindness.'[7]

Kitty Dukakis

Kitty Dukakis was born Katharine Dickson in Cambridge, Massachusetts in 1936. Jewish by birth and something of a radical, she dropped out of college to marry John Chaffetz when she was 19. The marriage didn't last after the birth of her son and she moved to Brookline, a Jewish area of Boston. She received her B.A. from Lesley College in 1963, the same year she married Michael Dukakis. She received a M.A. degree from Boston University School of Communication in 1982.

The 1988 presidential campaign of Michael Dukakis began when he announced his candidacy on March 16 1987, in a speech in Boston. He became the Democratic Party's nominee at the party's convention in Atlanta, Georgia on July 21, that year and lost the 1988 election to his Republican opponent, the sitting Vice President George H. W. Bush.

In 1989, Kitty was briefly hospitalized after drinking rubbing alcohol and in 1991, published her memoir, *Now You Know*, in which she discussed her drinking. The book also discussed the pressures of being a political wife. In the mid-'90s, she graduated from Boston University with a master's degree in Social Work. In 2002 she began a series of electroshocks having been inscribed with depression. Her brother-in-law Stelian had received electroshock as a college student, later talking of how unhelpful it had been.

Aged 80, Kitty Dukakis remains a leading advocate of the use of electroshock. With Larry Tye, a journalist, she wrote *Shock: The Healing Power of Electroconvulsive Therapy*.

A *New York Times* article suggests, 'Electroconvulsive therapy is not a one-and-done procedure. Mrs. Dukakis, 80, still receives maintenance treatment every seven or eight weeks. She said that she had minor memory lapses but that the treatment had banished her demons and that she no longer drank, smoked or took antidepressants.'[8] Dukakis receives her maintenance shock at McLean Hospital in Boston. McLean does about 10,000 such treatments a year on between 700 and 1000 people; in 1999, for example, there were 2,500 treatments.

Dukakis's psychiatrist is Charles Welch who appears promoting the benefits of electroshock on the MECTA video (see Vested interest and Vaslav Nijinsky). The

Times article includes links to an electroshock web-page hosted by the Dukakises and a 2014 NIMH study on electroshock in older people.[9]

Law and
Lou Reed

'The entire power of psychiatry is based on the commitment law ... What is crazy to one of us, is just funny or silly or cantankerous to another. The thought of losing one's liberty over one's deportment is a terrifying prospect.'[1]

Laws are made for those that make them rather than the public at large. The vested interest of politicians exposed daily to lobbyists and frequently financially backed by corporations ensures that laws and logic don't necessarily go hand in hand.[2]

For example, it has been said that half of us don't take the medications that the state wants us to (as prescribed by psychiatrists and general practitioners) and half takes drugs the state doesn't want us to (as sold by criminal drug dealers, traded in school play-grounds or bought online). The complex relationship between inscription, medication and the legality of certain dangerous drugs is summarised by Lenny Bruce, a comedian who used routines that included tales of his drug-taking and alcohol consumption:

'The big connections of the dangerous drugs are Squibb and Park-Lilly, Olin Mathison and Merc and Wyeth ... Dangerous drugs – that's the legal phrase – relates to all these ... mood elevators. They are not made in Guatemala, but in factories and for a purpose.'[3]

The law can be a blunt instrument. For example, English magistrates are bound by rules that mean that, whether or not someone can pay, she will be fined if she has not paid her TV licence. Three strikes and out; failure to pay after three fines means a custodial sentence – and she still owes for the unpaid licence.

In the UK, the 2007 Mental Health Act allows people to be formally detained in hospital in the interests of their own health or safety, or allows 'treatment' in the community and recall to hospital for assessment or treatment under a Community Treatment Order. The latest available figures show that the total number of detentions under The Act rose in 2016, increasing by 9 per cent to 63,622 compared to 58,399 detentions in 2014/15 This compares with an increase of 10 per cent between 2013/14 and 2014/15 and is the highest number since 2005/06 (43,361 detentions) a rise of just under fifty per cent over the period.

The use of section 136 of The Act increased by 18 per cent to 22,965. Section 136 legitimates people thought to be of danger to themselves or others being held in police cells for up to 24 hours before removal to a 'place of safety.' Police forces receive thousands of calls per annum from people threatening suicide, the majority of whom are known to services and not detained.

At the end of March 2016, 25,577 people were

subject to the Act, of whom 20,151 were detained in hospitals. There has been a continuing increase in the number of people detained in independent sector providers (ISPs) and in the proportion of all detained patients that they represent since NHS Digital started publishing the statistics in 2006.

On 31 March 2016, 5,954 people were being treated as detained patients in independent hospitals, representing 30 per cent of all detained patients on that day and the highest proportion since information was first made public on 31 March 2006, when 17 per cent of detained patients were in a private hospital.[4]

Asked in 1754 to undertake the supervision of private madhouses the English College of Physicians declined, in part because the idea was 'too troublesome' and because some members had vested interests in the institutions.[5] Eventually the Madhouse Act reached the statute books in 1774. Five commissioners, annually appointed by the College were to inspect madhouses within a seven mile radius of London and in the provinces a group of magistrates, accompanied by a doctor, fulfilled the same task.

The aim was to prevent illegal admission of the sane though there was no remit to explore the plight of other inmates. Pauper lunatics, who did not require medical certification for admittance were unprotected. It took until the Madhouse Act of 1828 to establish the Metropolitan Lunacy Commission with five doctors and up to 15 lay commissioners with the power to revoke or refuse to renew an asylum licence.[6]

After a report on the deplorable state of asylums in England and Wales the lunacy bills of 1845 led to the establishment of the Lunacy Commission that same year, this time with three legal and three medical professionals. For the upper and middle classes, certification was frequently suggested by family members. Reasons included wandering, violence to people or property, suicidality, 'delusions', 'foul language', and forms of 'moral insanity' involving women's sexual impropriety. Frances Willington, for example, was admitted to Ticehurst private asylum for 'labouring under nymphomania' while in 1847 Henrietta Golding was certified for her, 'inclinations to form an improper connection with a person of very inferior grade.'[7]

From the outset, commissioners and certifying doctors struggled with mutually incompatible notions of liberty. The position obtains today as industrialized societies such as the USA and UK fetishize individual freedom and individuality in the abstract; the much debated right of US citizens to carry guns is part of a discourse of liberty. At the same time, social mores consist of expectations to conformity in values and conduct.

The right to individual freedom may be suspended if the individual exercises that right by acting in ways disruptive to societal mores. Hence the Victorian paradox whereby many people were incarcerated after exercising their freedom to be different when the differences exceeded societal norms of propriety or in the case of violent acts, legal statute.

The paradox is still with us. Relatives will inscribe themselves and family members – especially children – and have those inscriptions confirmed by psy professionals if being 'different' is a threat to social status or property. Conversely, the possibility of obtaining state benefits through inscription means that people will enact 'insane' behaviour for entirely sane reasons in order to facilitate their 'right' to support. For some Victorian psychiatrists, appearing in court to justify their certification of certain patients these convolutions led to censure by the judiciary and the press:

'John Conolly, at that time England's best known consultant psychiatrist, was censured by ... Lord Chief Baron Sir Frederick Pollock ... and denounced ... for his apparent willingness to certify anyone of even mildly eccentric views or dissipated habits.'[8]

A century and a half later, it is a short step to someone being inscribed on spectrum 'disorders' such as schizophrenia, autism and, increasingly, bipolar.

Government is *of* the people rather than *for* the people. Broadly left-wing governments tend towards policies of protection and right wing governments towards control. Factors that promote 'health' might include a lack of pollution and the provision of safe places where children can play. Community and critical psychologists ally with policy-makers to promote a liberation philosophy though psy has declared these efforts as part of a primary prevention strategy in the field of so-called mental health to be like the Okenfenokee swamp, 'attractive from a distance, especially from the air, luring the unwary into quagmires and impenetrable by-ways.'[9]

Government ideology is implicit in the statute book. In 1933, the Prussian Ministry of Justice produced a memorandum on the admissibility of sterilization, eugenic abortion and the killing of people deemed of no value – those with 'incurable mental diseases.' In August 1939 the Reich Ministry of the Interior considered a change in the sterilization law and decreed the registration of children under three with a tribunal for hereditary diseases.[10] The tribunal selected 5,000 children with Down's Syndrome for extermination. The die was cast and legislation for the killing of 'degenerate' Jews and Bolsheviks duly followed (see Death-making and David Reville).

The history of psy's relationship to the law is replete with contradiction and ill-thought out consequences. In 1978, the Italian psychiatric reform act (Law 180) made institutionalisation of mad people illegal. On the face of it this was in response to the appalling state of existing asylums. Driven by the economic imperative psychiatric wards were instead established in general hospitals wherever psychiatric hospitals closed.

The outcome was that remaining and underfunded asylums became worse and: 'In some places the psychiatric wards in general hospitals ... produced some of the worst features of the old mental hospitals.' Proposed alternative services didn't develop leading to homes for elderly people and homeless hostels being

116

inundated.[11]

The outcome mirrored Szasz's analysis of the true status of the psychiatric population; in the absence of a family member to take them in, rather than 'ill', most publicly supported mental patients are unemployed, indigent and homeless. This has been the position since the first Poor Law in Britain. People are either poor through no fault of their own and (poorly) housed and (poorly) fed by the state (the origin of the workhouse) or they are poor through indigence and cast out to fend for themselves.

In Italy, politicians refused to pay for community care of people refused admission to hospitals and, once the hospitals were closed, turned a blind eye to increasing homelessness. Employability was key and jobs required a skilled and reliable workforce. Writing in *Libération* Franco Basaglia, a leading psychiatric reformer, said that the logic of the mental hospital had run its course.[12] Basaglia hadn't factored in economics.

For all its appearance of allying with left-wing ideals, the reform law was a long way from establishing better accommodation or employment for institutionalised patients and made no inroads towards Illich's 'Right to useful unemployment.'[13] Unsurprising, given the ways in which psy professions exist to *dis*able citizens through disparagement disguised as diagnosis, guesswork disguised as expertise and, as in the Italian example, a lack of understanding of wider social and economic factors.

Formal governance for psy in the first instance is an internalized Gaze (le Regard).[14] This might be positioned as 'conscience' though notions of good and bad are idiosyncratic and will reflect familial, professional and societal attitudes. Conduct can be justified by reference to expert authority, professional guidelines and regulations and notions of 'abnormality' or 'protecting the public.' Supervision, peer consultation and professional guidelines may change a professional's conduct or re-inforce it. In a context where members of psy exercise power over patients in, frequently, hidden settings (the consulting room or clinic, the electroshock suite, a ward side room) and informed consent is in the gift of the professional, that same professional can feel above the law and free to act in ways that appear arbitrarily cruel.

As noted in Assault and Antonin Artaud, it has frequently been suggested that legitimate psy interventions *constitute* cruelty. Beyond these normative interventions, psy has a history of innovative non-sanctioned methods that – to the outsider – hover around the edges of criminality whether via charging high fees for unsuccessful treatment or in the nature of such 'treatment'. The law can sometimes be used to challenge psy practice – with unpredictable con-sequences.

In 1877, for example, Forbes Winslow, a specialist in mental disorders, was sued for libel, assault, wrongful arrest, false imprisonment and trespass by a Mrs Weldon detained by Winslow in his private asylum in Hammersmith. The case led to a clause in the eventual 1890 Lunacy Act *giving legal protection to medical practitioners* who acted in good faith. The Act did not concern itself with treatment *per se* despite the efforts of reformers. Instead it focused on concerns about wrongful detention and systematised the need for medical certification for every compulsory admission with the exception of an 'urgency order' that allowed uncertified detention for up to seven days.[15]

In the USA, the legality or otherwise of psy interventions is decided upon differently in different States. For example, in 1973 Oregon passed legislation restricting psychosurgery (see Zealotry and Zelda Fitzgerald) to include the right to informed consent. California followed suit in 1976.[16]

John Rosen, a US psychiatrist specialising in 'therapy' of those inscribed as schizophrenic, was well known in the UK and US. Rosen published a critically acclaimed book on his methods which he summarised as 'beating.'[17] His second volume of collected papers received supportive reviews from eminent members of psy including Winnicott, Rogers, Searles, Fromm-Reichmann and Balint.[18] In 1971, Rosen won the Man of the Year award of the American Academy of Psychotherapy.

The Institute of Direct Analysis had been formed by Rosen in 1956 within the Department of Psychiatry at Temple University Medical Centre. Patients accused Rosen and his staff of rape and assault; one, Claudia Ehrman, was beaten to death by Karmen 'Jay' Patet, a 'therapist' who later pleaded guilty to manslaughter. The State Board of Medical Education and Licensure of the Department of the State of Pennsylvania accused Rosen of 67 violations of the Pennsylvania Medical

Practices Act and 35 violations of rules and regulations of the Medical Board.[19] To avoid trial he surrendered his licence in March, 1983.

One of John Rosen's protégées was Albert Honig who co-founded and became Medical Director of the Delaware County Mental Health Foundation in Doylestown, Pa. Honig oversaw the use of electric cattle prods and electric 'relaxicisors'. He was a doctor of osteopathy, his 'therapists' psychologists. An investigation by the Bucks County District Attorney's office found the therapists to be acting in 'good faith' (see above) and the 'treatments' legitimate. The report added that some patients had been suicidal and the Foundation represented a 'last chance' – the same rationale used by advocates of electroshock.

Interviewed in November 1986, Honig admitted that the cattle prods constituted a 'crazy' method but 'seemed to work.'[20] Honig became clinical professor in psychiatry at the Philadelphia College of Osteopathic Medicine and in 2009 published *The Insanity Wars,* a novel trailed as 'An original, adventurous, entertaining, humorous, amazing story of a young psychiatrist and his wife as their marriage is bombarded by the intense involvement with some of the world's sickest mentally ill.'[21] Honig was awarded 'Fellow of the Year' for the Association of Clinical Osteopathic Neuropsychiatric Physicians. He died in 2012.

In 1984, *Pulse* reported on a general practitioner working in Devon and then in London. One in seven patients were receiving electroshock for 'arthritis, indigestion, irritable bowel syndrome and aphthous ulcers.'[22]

In 1989, Gary Aden, founder and first president of the International Association for the Advancement of Electrotherapy (now The International Society for ECT and Neurostimulation) surrendered his licence after allegations of beating and having sex with patients. He branded two with heated metal devices, *including an iron that bore his initials.*'[23] (Original emphasis)

In Germany, a more direct use of electroshock *qua* brain assault has been used without sanction. '... [Dörner] recommends the use of electroshock for a situation when a 'therapist' is 'not able to engage in a sufficiently effective therapeutic alliance'. This is in order to produce 'someone suffering from an organic brain syndrome.'

For Dörner, this would bring relief to the patient as, 'A threat to life and limb makes psychotic anxiety superfluous.'[24]

In Texas, psychiatrists are obliged to report any deaths that occur within two weeks of electroshock. In the March-May quarter of 2007, Cypress Creek Hospital (see Research and Paul Robeson) reported one death (of a 22-year-old woman) occurring within two weeks of treatment. The woman's mother later sued the hospital.[25] Inscribed with bipolar disorder, post-traumatic stress disorder, and attention deficit hyperactivity disorder, the patient had been determined to be a suicide risk and was voluntarily admitted to Cypress Creek at the end of April 2007. Her prescribed drugs included Effexor XR, Eskalith, Adderall, Campral, Zyprexa, Provera, Topamax, and Xanax. After admission electroshock and Ambien CR were added to this regimen.

On May 2, she was prescribed hydrocodone for pain from a knee injury and on May 3, she was also prescribed Oxycontin. During the early hours of the following morning she was found to have no pulse and was declared dead at 3.04 am. Toxicology results showed that she died as a result of Zyprexa toxicity.

The case brought against Cypress Creek Hospital by the mother was thrown out of court because the author of the litigant's expert-report was not a physician.[26] A usual response to this from an activist perspective might be something along the lines: 'Another tragic case of a life lost through the iniquity of big bad Pharma in alliance with psychiatry.'

Such a response positions the patient and her mother as trusting innocents in the face of cynically exploitative efforts of psy. A rejoinder might be: 'Have these women been living in a cave for thirty years? Do they know nothing of the growing criticism towards so called experts in everything from weather-forecasting to bankers? And what in G-d's name did a woman think that *nine* psychotropics would do to her in a world where the television, diet magazines, vegans, vegetarians and neighbours, friends and family on a host of dietary regimes must have warned her of the ills inherent in what we ingest?'

Are we to believe that two twenty-first century women were really that cut-off when a quick check on Google for adverse effects would have been informative? It is a common defence that patients 'weren't to know' of the adverse effects of drugs, a claim that simultaneously places the responsibility at the manufacturer's door and renders the claimant a naïve victim.

Some patients are more canny: 'A second spell in hospital followed, where my consultant wanted to try electroconvulsive therapy, but I had seen *One Flew Over the Cuckoo's Nest* ... I flatly refused because someone else on the ward had had it and he could hardly remember anything at all since ...'[27]

French, English and US courts of the nineteenth century witnessed alienists and psychiatrists struggling for ascendancy and the right to judge the mentality of the accused and the possibility of claiming insanity as a defence (see Precision and Mervyn Peake). For half a century, accused persons have claimed versions of insanity as mitigation for crimes from petty theft to murder and called on psy professionals for help.

The current ascendancy of psy in the law and public consciousness, however, is not always confirmed as justified in more probing analyses: 'Years of experience for psy experts do not improve the standards of their testimony and a reliance on anecdote to support testimony is inaccurate and unscientific.'[28] The author of the quote, David Stein, suggests so called psy expertise is, in any case, predicated '...on a career of doing nothing but *junk science*.'[29] (original emphasis).

Despite such concerns expert witnesses from psy operating as instruments of the law use the rhetorical devise of persuasion through obfuscation and a battery of psychometric tests to help condemn, excuse or reward (via compensation for injury) claimants, litigants and the accused. For example, *The Times* reports on the 'divisibility' notion in relation to legal claims for 'psychiatric injury' in a case involving the UK's Court of Appeal in which an employment tribunal was trying to ascertain how to apportion harm suffered via the employer's wrong-doing and that which may have been due to other causes. In this particular case a woman's claim for perceived harm caused by sex discrimination rested on suffering which, quite reasonably, could have been seen as arising from circumstances unconnected with the claimed sex discrimination. A 'discount' could be applied if the claimant was seen – by expert testimony – to 'have' a 'vulnerable personality.'[30]

'Vulnerability' is, however, contextual. A child is not 'vulnerable' to assault in the company of respectful adults although there seems confusion around the possibility that assaultive men can be 'vulnerable' to women in 'alluring' clothing. For psychiatric patients with experience of the professional or institutional gaze, a vulnerability and realistic wariness may be an outcome. For example, as part of a system for monitoring praxis at Shelton psychiatric hospital in Shrewsbury voluntary Patients' Council members visited the wards to discuss the regime with patients one of whom said: 'If I complain, they will probably give me an injection.'[31] Complaints at Ashworth Special Hospital in Liverpool led to two public inquiries; both suggested hospital closure. Instead, the outer wall was built higher.[32]

The American Food and Drug Association regulates drugs and devices in the US. Electroshock devices come under the purview of the Neurological Devices Panel and are placed in one of three risk categories. Despite recording thousands of complaints and concerns about electroshock, neither the American Food and Drug Association nor electroshock pressure groups achieved the reclassification of shock machines as Class III (High risk) medical devices which must be proven safe before their use until 1976.

The shock machines were classified Class III for 'depression (unipolar and bipolar), schizophrenia, bipolar manic (and mixed) states, schizoaffective disorder and schizophreniform disorder.' In 2011, the FDA Advisory Panel advised that use for those inscribed with catatonia would be down-graded to Class 2. All other uses remained at Class 3; the psychiatrists had voted for Class 2, the psychologists and neurologists for Class 3.[33] In 2014, the American Psychiatric Association launched a petition to reclassify electroshock as a low-risk treatment.

In itself this was something of an exercise in illusion; the list of 'disorders' implies their existence as entities rather than linguistic constructs. As noted in Inscription and Insulin coma this sleight of hand has had its critics since the beginnings of modern psychiatry. In 1835 James Cowles Prichard used an appendix in his *Treatise on Insanity* to examine French alienists' attempts to correlate brain pathology with mad behaviour. He concluded that there 'were simply too many instances where overt insanity could not be correlated with structural abnormalities.'[34]

The situation hasn't changed – indeed could never change due to the metaphorical nature of so called psychiatric disorder – but this does not hinder those who prescribe electroshock. Insanity appears to have no physical correlates yet for sanity to be achieved a physically powerful shock to the brain is seen as necessary.

Advocates acknowledge that they 'don't know how electroshock works.' If disorders cannot be located in the brain and the action of electroshock is generally unknown a consent form need simply say: 'You have a non-physical imaginary illness. We shall treat you with a physical treatment but we can't imagine why it might work.'

Laws in different countries and states are applied in different ways and contested in different ways. For example, The Law Project for Psychiatric Rights (PsychRights.Org) was, until recently, a public interest law firm maintaining a strategic legal campaign against forced psychiatric drugging and electroshock in the United States. The Law Project suggests United States' law, where people's right to the least restrictive (in the case of psychiatric incarceration) or least intrusive (in the case of forced drugging or electroshock) alternatives, is violated as a matter of course.

In law, people in the United States have the right to the least intrusive alternatives before forced drugging or electroshock can be ordered by a court. In Alaska (where the Law Project survives with reduced energy for campaigning), this has been interpreted to mean that if there is a feasible less intrusive alternative to forced drugging, the state has to either provide it or let the person go. As part of the Project's activities the PsychRights website is instructive. For example, it cites research indicating that psychiatric drugs (and electroshock) are very harmful without any real benefit for most of the people taking them; people diagnosed with serious mental illness in the public mental health system in the United States have a life span that is 25 years shorter than that of the general population.[35] After the first neuroleptic, chlorpromazine (Thorazine in the United States, Largactil in the UK), and the other phenothiazines, such as Haldol, Mellaril, and Stelazine, were introduced in the 1950s, people's life spans were decreased by 10–15 years. The second generation of neuroleptics and the increasing use of polypharmacy have brought early death forward by another decade.[36]

In a landmark case in 2006, a South Carolina woman was awarded $635,177 after successfully suing her psychiatrist for referring her for electroshock; the procedure had cost her all memories of the man to whom she had been married for thirty years. Her legal victory was unique; since the first legal case for shock induced memory loss in 1974 there were a number of out of court settlements but this was the first time a judge ruled in favour of a shock survivor.[37]

Private madhouses and public asylums in the UK and epileptic colonies, asylums, and psychiatric clinics in the US were (and to an extent, remain) places of experimentation where psychiatrists tried their latest interventions on a captive population. Consent to treatment was either not seen as relevant, given by relatives, taken-for granted if the patient was voluntary or, subsumed within a rhetorical 'greater good' as patients became guinea pigs. In psychiatric legislation consent is a potential contract between the state and the person.

In England and Wales, the Mental Health Act 1983 allowed the use of electroshock on detained patients whether or not they had capacity to consent to it. Following amendments in 2009, electroshock could not generally be given to a patient with capacity who refuses it, irrespective of his or her detention under the Act. Even if a patient is deemed to lack capacity, if he or she makes a valid advance decision refusing shock then they should not be given it.

If they do not have an advance decision, the psychiatrist must obtain an independent second opinion (which is also the case if the patient is under the age of consent). There is an exception regardless of consent and capacity; under Section 62 of the Act, if the treating psychiatrist says the need for treatment is urgent they may start a course of electroshock without authorization.

From 2003 to 2005, about 2,000 people a year in England and Wales were treated without their consent under the Mental Health Act. Concerns have been raised by the official regulator that psychiatrists are too readily assuming that patients have the capacity to consent to their treatments, and that there is a worrying lack of independent advocacy. In Scotland, the Mental Health (Care and Treatment) (Scotland) Act 2003 also gives patients with capacity the right to refuse shock. In one of the few jurisdictions where recent statistics on electroshock usage are available, a national audit by the Scottish ECT Accreditation Network indicated that 77 per cent of patients who received shock in 2008 were capable of giving informed consent.[38]

Some activists, unimpressed by the psychiatric drive for acceptance as bona fide medical doctors, have pressed for changes in the law. For adults in Europe electroshock is illegal only in Slovenia. Germany has ratified the use of advance directives.[39] To that extent Europeans are only safe from electroshock in Slovenia (where psychiatrists continue to refer potential recipients over the border to Croatia) or, as German citizens, if they have signed an advance directive stating they do not want to receive electroshock in Germany.

Other survivors have suggested questions concerning compulsion worthy of research: What are the longer-term effects of forced interventions and coercive treatments? How does coercion affect compliance? Is there an increase in non-compliance after patients have been coerced? Is there an increase in treatment avoidance among people who have been coerced? For their part psy professional allies with research experience might offer 'advice, consultation and expertise in helping research findings reach a broader audience.'[40]

The relationship of psy to the law is complex, constantly under review and critique and a source of income for many and despair for at least the same number. For Szasz: 'The practice of psychiatry rests on

129

two pillars: mental illness and involuntary mental hospitalization. Each of these elements justifies and reinforces the other.'[41] Szasz has described institutional psychiatry as a form of slavery – quite literally in the case of asylum inmates who worked for negligible reward as gardeners, ground-staff and hospital attendants from the mid nineteenth century to the late twentieth.[42]

Szasz notes that, since the *Donaldson* case of 1975 patients incarcerated in US psychiatric hospitals but not treated have been unconstitutionally deprived of their liberty.[43] A licensed psy professional who does not 'treat' a person already deprived of their liberty through involuntary committal can be sued by the patient for denying the right to treatment.

This might appear to bring us into the presence of the red queen in *Alice Through the Looking Glass*. Kelley, however, discusses a law suit brought by the patient of a psychotherapeutically inclined institution (Chestnut Lodge) because the treating psychiatrist *didn't* prescribe medication after the patient had been inscribed with three different types of depression (the opinion of the co-ordinating psychiatrist was that the patient suffered from 'pathological narcissism').[44]

There is an ever-shifting interplay between the law and psy. Governments make laws and psy professionals are bound by them as citizens. In their professional practice they can use mental health legislation to deprive fellow citizens of their liberty and enforce treatment. In Italy and elsewhere those same psy professionals – as part of a de-institutionalisation movement – deprived patients of places to live. The law simultaneously defends the right to liberty while curtailing that right for people who are seen as a threat to themselves, others or property. Psy survivors and activists have urged change in laws on forced treatment and demanded more transparency to allow informed consent. In court members of psy have been vilified as charlatans and called on as experts.

Patients have use psy practitioners in court and sue them for harm or inappropriate treatment and assault. Psy professionals claim to be able to detect if someone should avoid the criminal justice system on the grounds of 'mental illness' or be excused their criminal conduct due to 'depression' or 'trauma.' Convoluted legal rituals for psy professionals, recipients, judges, magistrates and activists continue to attract a critical gaze.

Lou Reed

In 1951, Sam Phillips, the young founder of Sun Records, produced *Rocket 88* for a band called Jackie Brenston and his Delta cats – but only because Phillips thought the saxophonist (Brenston) was a better singer than their vocalist, Ike Turner.

Rocket 88 has been called the first rock 'n' roll record. Released via Chess Records it sold half a million copies. Two months later, aged 27 Phillips had a breakdown and was electro-shocked for the second time; the first had been when he was twenty. He recovered after what he described as 'bibliotherapy' and went on to launch radio station WHER in 1955.[45] It was the first all-female radio station in the United States, as almost every position at the station was held by a woman. Phillips was not the first, nor will he be the last, member of the music industry to be electro-shocked.

Like many others, I first began to really appreciate Lou Reed in the early 1970s post-Velvet Undergound; *Transformer*. Since then, the awesome *Metal Machine Music,* the harrowing *Berlin* and the beautiful *New York* and *Songs for Drella* have come and gone. *Perfect Day* even crops up, in full ironic vein in *Trainspotting*. But that's not why Lou appears here.

Creedmoor State Psychiatric Hospital (see Bystanders and Bud Powell) in Queens, New York opened in 1912 in Queen's Village as a farm colony for the nearby Brooklyn State Hospital, originally for 32 patients. In the 1960s hundreds of children diagnosed with 'autistic schizophrenia' were given electroshock there.

Lou Reed's parents had sent him for 24 sessions at two day intervals during the summer of 1959 because he was up and down and rebellious. His mother denied the admission had anything to do with his sexuality. Reed said that Creedmoor was 'hell.'

Marketing
and Movies

There is a discernible 'evolution' in physical treatments for the mad. Underlying the change, a pattern can be detected whereby new approaches are heralded as 'breakthroughs'.

As in the marketing of any product, the faults of the previous product are emphasised and the (frequently known) adverse effects of the newest venture downplayed. The fundamental problem that all so-called conditions are linguistic constructions (see Inscription and Insulin coma) is ignored in marketing campaigns – rather like ignoring the carbon footprint in the manufacturing process of 'green' automobiles (or the fact it is greener to walk, cycle or take the bus).

For the psy industry, drug names are carefully selected – 'Valium' suggests becoming valiant, 'Librium' was to liberate the recipient and so on. Therapies are similarly branded, three-letter acronyms being popular. 'Electrocution' has less market appeal than electroshock but 'electro-convulsive therapy' captures the magical 'therapy' trope and is usually transcribed as a market-friendly three letter acronym – ECT.

Earlier marketing campaigns for electroshock mirrored those for psycho-tropics. Photographs of, usually female, patients before and after a particular intervention regularly appeared in medical journals whose publishers also continue to benefit from manufacturers' promotional budgets. Before the intervention the person appears sad and is dowdily dressed. After, a smiling house-wife is shown complete with smiling children.

These images reflect a little discussed dynamic within psychiatric discourse. It frequently emerges that the partners and spouses of famous folk are subjected to silencing regimes of moral orthopaedics such as incarceration and 'treatment.' In 1839, for example, Rosina Bulwer-Lytton, wife of the novelist Edward Bulwer Lytton published *Cheveley, or the Man of Honour*. It was a near-libellous fiction satirising her husband's alleged hypocrisy.[1]

In June 1858, when her husband was standing as parliamentary candidate for Hertfordshire, she denounced him at the hustings. He retaliated by denying her access to her children and withdrawing her allowance. He then had her committed to an asylum. Following a public outcry, she was released a few weeks later. Rosina was made of stern stuff and chronicled her incarceration in her memoir, *A Blighted Life,* published in 1880.[2] (see also Zealotry and Zelda Fitzgerald)

For the spouses and parents of many less well known women and children, however, incarceration and electroshock is a route to a peaceful life. Acquiescence to abusive authority is frequently an outcome of punishment (see Torture).

For men or parents who find domestic life more turbulent than they can tolerate the inherent punishment of psychiatric intervention for spouses or children who refuse to be subjugated is always an option.

Electroshock, if mentioned at all by groups or individuals with little vested interest (for or against), generally has a bad, sometimes alarmist, press. A negative public and recipient reaction to what is seen as harmful praxis thus requires a remarketing of physical assault by psy practitioners and the associated publishing industry.

The marketing of depression as a condition goes hand in hand with the marketing of a host of treatments, both 'psychological' and physical. For example, a recent article in *The Lancet* claims that a review of 21 named anti-depressants over almost four decades showed all of them to be 'effective' and suggests 'at least a million more Britons' should be prescribed ('put on') them. The review states that too many GPs are 'squeamish' about their use – despite acknowledging that the UK has the fourth highest prescription rate in the West. Depression is described as a 'disorder' and compared to cancer.[3]

For those inscribed as depressed electroshock has always been marketed as 'safe' and 'effective.' The Royal College of Psychiatrists *ECT Handbook* suggests using the words as part of the response to any concerns (see Evidence and Electrocution). Jones and Baldwin, however, remark in an article from over 20 years ago:

'ECT has been repackaged in a manner designed to censor public opinion. Empirical research, based on adequate methodological data, does not exist ...'[4]

The 'repackaging' of electroshock has a ready audience. In a service culture dominated by demands for efficiency and cost saving, electroshock can be offered as an efficient means of processing patients if waiting lists for psychological therapies are extensive, resources (hospital beds for example) at a premium and pharmacology (usually the first recommended treatment) has failed.

Further, in a litigious culture, given the claim that electroshock is a 'life-saver' (often backed up by recipient testimony), *not* suggesting it can be regarded as risky if the patient is suicidal (see Law and Lou Reed).

Thus, factors outwith the nature of recipients' alleged difficulties or context of their distress take precedence when making treatment proposals. For the psychiatrist the ability to tolerate fear and existing preferences for non-physical interventions in the work context are important as potential ways for patients to avoid electroshock. Equally, a litigious-aware psychiatrist working in a context where electroshock is regularly used is more likely to recommend the procedure, especially if colleagues are passionate about it (see Zealotry and Zelda Fitzgerald). More overt marketing or rebranding is unnecessary in pro-electroshock psychiatric contexts.

Despite that, the repackaging and marketing of electroshock continues. In the UK, it is predominantly confined to older women, performed with the consent of relatives or with the approval of second opinion doctors. Any 'controversy' is limited by the lack of publicity for the praxis and its invisibility within the clinic. Relatives usually need to be reasonably certain that electroshock is the best option and the power (for good as well as ill) of psy professionals is increased if they can give examples of successful past interventions; not dissimilar to a car salesperson with tales of happy customers. Any debate concerning electroshocking children and adolescents is mostly confined to anti-electroshock activists, frequently online, and within the pages of psychiatric journals. These are resources not open to many parents who thus depend on the 'expert' in front of them. The wish – unconscious or conscious – held by family members to punish the prospective recipient (see above) can complement an electroshock preference held by the professional. Such a wish makes a forceful sales technique unnecessary.

Research articles and reviews of electroshock are almost comedic in their repetition of the terms 'safe' and 'effective'. A cynic might be tempted to ask why researchers need to repeat these key words so often. Perhaps researchers are trying to convince themselves that electrocuting a child is a perfectly normal thing to do.

The repetition echoes the warning given to the character played by Cameron Diaz in *Knight and Day*: 'If someone says to trust him and you are going to be safe, run, they are probably going to kill you.'[5]

The promotional campaign for electroshock is not limited to the public as many professionals remain ignorant of its use. A paper in the *Journal of Electroconvulsive Therapy* examined the knowledge, experience and attitudes towards the use of electroconvulsive treatment in minors among child and adolescent psychiatrists and psychologists. A majority of the respondents said they had minimal knowledge about the use of electroshock in children and adolescents. Lack of confidence in providing a second opinion was reported by three-quarters of respondents. The majority regarded electroshock as a treatment of last resort. Compared with those with minimal knowledge, respondents with 'advanced knowledge' reported a higher perception of safety and efficacy, perhaps unsurprising given the constant repetition of the 'safe and effective' claim.[6]

Sham electroshock literature supports the conclusions that real electroshock 'is no more effective than placebo, except during the period of time the ECT is being administered; even that difference is modest; a modest amount of cost is required for the overall cost-benefit of ECT to be negative; and, the effectiveness of ECT is over-endorsed repeatedly.'[7]

The Royal College of Psychiatrists prefers to state: 'Although a *safe and effective treatment*, ECT remains controversial,'[8] (my italics) and continues, 'In placebo ECT, the patient has exactly the same things done to them – including going to the ECT rooms and having the anaesthetic and muscle relaxant – but no electrical current is passed and there is no fit. In these studies, the patients who had standard ECT were much more likely to recover, and did so more quickly than those who had the placebo treatment.'[9] This position ignores the widely held view that – whatever the damaging effects to the brain of electrocution – there is a low, but real risk of death during electroshock due to the anaesthesia. The Canadian Psychiatric Association underlines efficacy and safety: 'When used properly, ECT is a *safe and effective treatment* which should continue to be available as a therapeutic option for the treatment of mental disorders.'[10] (My emphasis.) Publishers too have a vested interest in promotional exercises by electroshock proponents; in 2013 Oxford University Press published *Electroconvulsive Therapy in Children and Adolescents.*[11]

Writing in *The Independent,* George Kirov cites the ECT Accreditation Service (ECTAS): 'The data is (sic) freely available on the Royal College of Psychiatrists website and counted 2,148 courses of ECT given during 2014-2015. A quick glance through the ECTAS document can tell us a lot about the nature of the illnesses treated with ECT and the remarkable outcomes: 51.7 per cent of people were rated as 'severely ill' and another 18.7 per cent as 'among the most severely ill' prior to ECT. At the end of their treatment, however, 74.4 per cent were 'much improved/very much improved', while only 1.7 per cent had deteriorated. This is a treatment reserved for the most severely depressed patients, and it produces unrivalled improvements.'

Kirov cites a report from 2004 before asking: 'And does anybody really think that if we can't explain why something works, we should not use it? That would mean not using many of the pharmaceuticals on the market today. Drugs regulators, such as the US Food and Drug Administration, only require that a pharmaceuticals firm proves the efficacy of a drug, not provide definitive evidence for how it works.'[12]

The article moves from suggesting that electroshock is 'unrivalled' to the empirical process of modern medicine dismissing any dissent by appeals to pragmatism. As its likely audience will have been willing pharmaceutical guinea pigs for some time, he is preaching to the converted.

The pro-electroshock lobby is further aided by recipients who use the modern version of the movies (Facebook) to promote shock. The byline for a recent clip reads:

'There are a lot of myths surrounding ECT for medication resistant depression. I considered ECT the last resort for treating my depression. I have medication resistant depression. With Bipolar 1, the mania and depression cycles severely affect me. Having ECT gave me an option to live a normal life again rather than choosing the dark, hopeless pit of despair. I hope you find this video useful.'[13]

And the movies...

From Lang's *M*, via Bunuel's *The Exterminating Angel* and Powell and Pressburger's *The Red Shoes,* to Kurosowa's *Ran,* directors have portrayed forms of madness, frequently with violent protagonists (for example, Jack Nicholson in *The Shining*). Associating madness and violence has been a theme in the media for over a century.

Other directors have offered a more nuanced perspective. Olivia de Havilland starred in Anatole Litvak's *The Snake Pit* (1948), a chronicle of a woman's stay in a psychiatric hospital. Kazan's *A Streetcar Named Desire* stars Vivien Leigh as Blanche DuBois who moves in with her sister in New Orleans and is tormented by her brutish brother-in-law while her reality crumbles. Leigh herself was notoriously difficult to work with. For much of her adult life, she was inscribed with manic depression and had recurrent bouts of chronic tuberculosis, first diagnosed in the mid-1940s. She died of TB at the age of 53.

Bergman's 1961 *Through a Glass Darkly* tells the story of a young woman inscribed with schizophrenia who spends time with her family on a remote island having delusions about meeting G-d, who appears to her in the form of a monstrous spider.

In Sam Fuller's 1963 *Shock Corridor,* a journalist convinces a psychiatrist to coach him to appear insane; this involves relating imaginary accounts of incest with his 'sister', impersonated by his exotic-dancer girlfriend. Locked up in the institution where the murder took place, he begins to go mad. After a hospital riot he is straitjacketed and subjected to electroshock. He begins imagining that his girlfriend really is his sister, and after violently extracting a confession from the killer writes his story. Broken, he has to stay in the hospital for an undefined period. The film pre-dates by a decade Rosenhan's famous experiment demonstrating that conduct in mad places is invariably seen as typical of inscribed inmates.[14]

Although Rosenhan demonstrated the biased perspective of staff taking notes on his play-acting 'patients' the research shows that it is equally possible to conclude that the mad identities of the existing patients were being constructed by the psychiatric panopticon (see Governmentality and Gene Tierney). In turn, the conduct of the patients can be regarded as a function of the way in which people *become* their environment – subject a person in a locked ward to constant scrutiny by those in authority and that person soon shows all the signs of 'paranoia.'

They Might Be Giants, made in 1971, starred George C. Scott as a millionaire who retreats into fantasy after his wife's death, imagining himself to be Sherlock Holmes. Wearing a deerstalker and complete with pipe and violin, he spends his days in a homemade criminal laboratory, constantly paranoid about Moriarty. His brother (played by Lester Rawlins) tries to place Justin under observation in a mental institution so he can get power of attorney and attracts the attention of Dr Mildred Watson (played by Joanne Woodward), a psychiatrist. Initially dismissive of Watson's attempts to psychoanalyze him, he incorporates her into his life as Doctor Watson to his Holmes.[15]

They Might Be Giants takes its title from a quote from a quote in *Don Quixote* – another tale of inspiration disguised as madness.

One Flew Over the Cuckoo's Nest (1975) and *Frances* (1982) deal with what filmmakers imagined –

for Andrew Scull – as the 'shock 'em and mutilate 'em brigade of biological psychiatrists.' In Scull's review of cinema's depiction of madness at the movies, he says that the first fifty years were dominated by psychoanalysis: 'But it was biology not psychology that would soon triumph.'[16]

Frances stars Jessica Lange as actress Frances Farmer (see Fits and Frances Farmer). The film chronicles Farmer's life from high school student to her short lived film career in the 1930s, her 1940s' psychiatric institutionalization and eventual deinstitutionalization in the 1950s. The film was advertised as a true account of Farmer's life but the script has been criticised for its invention and sensationalization. In particular, the film depicts Farmer as having been lobotomized. Breggin has claimed that electroshock is an electric lobotomy; though Farmer was repeatedly drugged and shocked, she did not literally undergo a lobotomy.[17]

An inherent problem with filmic accounts based on 'a true story' is that a retelling of real events is not considered sufficiently dramatic. For Farmer, the simple truth would have been more than enough for most audiences.

In the HBO (TV) series *Six Feet Under* season 5, George undergoes electroshock to deal with his increasing paranoia. The depiction is shown realistically, with an actual shock machine.

Jane Campion's *An Angel at My Table* fictionalizes the experiences of author and poet Janet Frame (see: Justification and Janet Frame). Released from an asylum, 'Karin' rejoins her cold and distant family. Reality slips as she believes she is being visited by G-d.

Movies are not bound to tell the truth. Even in still photographs, 'the camera always lies', though for many the depiction of events on nightly news bulletins is more persuasive than printed text. In the motion picture industry cars, clothes, idioms of speech, even street signs can be shown as exiting long before they were invented.

Clint Eastwood directed *Changeling* in 2008. It tells the story of a woman whose drive to independence threatens those around her, especially men. Deemed unmanageable and labelled hysterical, she is forced into an institution and electroshocked. Although her fate mirrors that of countless women, the film's setting of 1928 predates Cerletti's first use of electroshock by a decade. The film has echoes of the injustice and cruelty foisted on Jack Nicholson's McMurphy in 1975's *One Flew Over the Cuckoo's Nest*. An essential difference is that in the latter film the evils of institutional authority are embodied in the character of a woman – Nurse Ratched (played by Louise Fletcher).

This gender reversal whereby the female protagonist is represented as bad via 'male' gender stereotypes (Ratched is full of bottled-up rage which explodes into vengeance after McMurphy attacks her) is noted by Karlene Faith as typical of fictional representations of female aggressors.[18] Electroshocked, McMurphy fakes brain damage before saying he is even more fired up. His ultimate fate? Lobotomy. Though ostensibly fiction, the film charts a steady progression for many patients during the 1950s; incarceration and drugs are followed by insulin coma and electroshock and finally lobotomy, sometimes several times.

Mark Rapley has argued that 'on message' portrayals of 'mental disorder', not infrequently in the form of biopics, secure contemporary popular recognition for supposedly 'true' depictions of inscribable madness. He cites 'films such as *Rain Man* (Autism) - Academy Award for Best Film, 1988; *As Good as it Gets* (Obsessive Compulsive Disorder) - Academy Awards for Best Actor and Best Actress, 1997; *A Beautiful Mind* (Paranoid schizophrenia) - Academy Awards for Best Picture, Best Director, Best Adapted Screenplay, and Best Actress in a Supporting Role, 2001; *Girl, Interrupted* (Borderline Personality Disorder) - Academy Award for Best Supporting Actress, 1999; 1990's *The Shining* ('psycho killer') and *The Silence of the Lambs* (criminally insane serial killer) – 'Big Five' Academy Award Winner, 1991.'[19] In each case, the so-called illness is effectively marketed, a move described as 'disease-mongering.'[20]

Normality
and Novels

Naming conduct as 'problems' is part of the disciplining process wherein 'normality' (actually behaviour which is useful for the maintenance of power in society) is defined by default.[1] Someone undressing in a café is likely to disrupt the sale of coffee and amuse or disturb the clientele and staff. If the police are called, the person may then be seen by a duty psychiatrist who, with few other options, may place the person in a psychiatric ward (if a bed is available). Order will have been restored and the café can go about its business.

For a child bored in a class-room, understandable conduct such as staring out of the window or disrupting the class may be inscribed as Attention Deficit Hyperactivity Disorder (ADHD). Ritalin or a similar drug will sufficiently dull the child such that 'normal' schooling can continue for the entire class. 'Normality' in both examples is any conduct that does not disrupt the social order.

As a feature of governmentality (see Governmentality and Gene Tierney) the 'norm' loses any statistical meaning and becomes instead a way for people to be judged and to monitor their own behaviour. The mythical happy married couple with two children may feature on social media such as Facebook but only exists as a normality-defining cliché, one that the over-whelming majority of the global population has never experienced. In comparing ourselves to these tropes, ordinary people can develop a sense of failure, something to be ameliorated through counselling, therapy or toeing the conservative line.

'Normality' is better read as desirability. It may be normal to be unhappy, paid the minimum wage for boring work, pre-occupied with concerns about relationships, body image and a lack of money potentially leading to a request to be psychiatrically inscribed in order to receive medication and state benefit payments but none of these things are desirable. We are disciplined to value happiness, well-paid work, reciprocally beneficial relationships predicated on stereotypical images of attractiveness – all desirable in a modern, consumerist context.[2]

In times of war, 'normality' implies patriotism and an aversion to 'the enemy.' Szasz remarks that during World War Two, psycho-analysts – many of whom were refugees from Nazi Germany – were employed by the military to explain why thousands of soldiers were unwilling to die for their country. Psychiatrists 'spouting psychoanalytic jargon' were valued for their 'arcane knowledge and patriotism.' He goes on:

'But it was all show, devoid of substance. Chairmen of psychiatry departments in medical schools, directors of state hospitals, and psychiatrists who used ECT (Electroconvulsive therapy) on their patients all displayed psychoanalytic credentials...'[3]

He doesn't add that some notable analytic group theorists (for example, Foulkes and Bion) had themselves been officers in the First World War and were responsible for theories that directly reflected their position as officers while simultaneously ignoring the power imbalances within military group therapy sessions.

The new normality is the ubiquity of the Web, Facebook and the app explosion. Psy has been quick on the uptake providing a world of inventive fun for boys and girls with toys. Vasan claims there are now 10,000 mental health apps.[4] Digital psychiatry is, we are told, the future.[5] For Vasan 'notable events' in 2017 included Google offering the public the PHQ-9 depression screening scale. When Internet users are searching for depression, a completed PHQ-9 will next redirect the person, with a screening score, to the National Alliance of Mental Illness (NAMI) website. The Google app begins:

'*Editor's note:*

Now when you search for 'clinical depression' on Google on mobile, you'll see a Knowledge Panel that will give you the option to tap 'check if you're clinically depressed', which will bring you to PHQ-9, a clinically validated screening questionnaire to test what your likely level of depression may be. To ensure that the information shared in the PHQ-9 questionnaire is accurate and useful, we have partnered with the National Alliance on Mental Illness on this announcement.'[6]

NAMI claims that depression is 'A brain disorder [and]... abnormal neural activity may be the cause.' Like Australia's SANE and similar family, carer and patient organizations, NAMI receives considerable funding from pharmaceutical companies (see Vested interest and Vaslav Nijinsky).

Meanwhile, the *Psychiatric Times* continues to define normality by default. Daily articles feature supposed 'cures' and 'breakthroughs' for schizophrenia, depression and dementia. The breakthroughs are always technical praxis, never simple things like being kind or generous to patients and no acknowledgement that hearing voices, feeling low or losing your marbles might be part of ordinary life. In an overwhelmingly American view of the 'norm', no-one is expected to find internal voices more interesting than television, discover that life without love is pointless however many possessions one has or – in the absence of stimulation and friendship – realize that gradually opting out through dementia is preferable to loneliness.

Enshrined in the Constitution, the right to the pursuit of happiness (by gun-owning protection of property) doesn't acknowledge the happiness to be found by pretending madness. The *Psychiatric Times* prefers a version of reality that depicts sanity (in an insane world) as inscribable and the human condition (a constant struggle for meaning) as abnormal.[7]

An article in the online version promotes the new normality of virtual electronic/digital communication that mimics conversation and psychotherapy. The Chatbot is a computer algorithm that uses artificial intelligence to simulate human conversation with patients in a way that is meant to be therapeutic. Just as bots can be used to help people make online purchases, it is suggested they can be trained to understand emotional responses and react accordingly. So far, Chatbots have found a wide range of uses, from delivering cognitive behaviour therapy for people who self-inscribe as depressed or anxious to reaching out to refugees in Syria.

Literary diversions

From Homer, Catullus and his homoerotic poetry, through Chaucer to Dickens and J.K. Rowling, writers have attempted to portray life in all its vicissitudes. All describe longing, lust, wandering, wondering and the struggle for meaning without once invoking psy inscription. Convinced by the new science of genetics, Zola's *Les Rougon-Macquart* series of novels explore the power of 'natural' evil passed on through generations. The more earthly (and poorer until sponsored by a countess) Balzac wrote convincingly of avarice and the terror of debt in *La Comedie Humaine*. Alienism was in its infancy; neither novelist required a psy expert to give them opinions on madness and the farcical nature of life.[8]

Jonathan Swift, who had been declared of unsound mind in 1742, died in 1745. Twelve years later, his bequest of eleven thousand pounds (an extraordinary amount of money at the time) enabled with additional funds the city of Dublin to open St. Patrick's Hospital. Now re-named St. Patrick's University Hospital, it claims to offer twelve per cent of Ireland's 'in-patient care and treatment needs.'[9]

Swift would have been a candidate for admission in admitting that he was an 'incurable scribbler'.[10] His satirical view of madness contrasted with his bequest to manage the mad. He viewed madness as a position with method – closer to laziness and revenge against loved ones than a loss of reason. In *A Tale of a Tub,* he describes a madman (the tailor) as '... run made with pride.' Pride, rather than lack of reason, is the cause of the tailor's insanity.[11]

Zola was inscribed as a result of his writings: perhaps, had electroshock been prescribed he would, like David Foster Wallace, have received it. Foster Wallace (author of *Infinite Jest a*nd *The Pale King*) was first electroshocked as a teenager. It went on for many years before his suicide aged 46.

Elizabeth Gaskell's father, John, was a factory hand addicted to opium. She had originally intended *Mary Barton* to be called *John Barton*. In the novel, the depiction of the poverty and exploitation in industrial Manchester (described with cruel realism in Engels' *The Condition of the Working Class in England*) makes opium an understandable escape. John is a victim of his social conditions and the loss of his beloved wife. In the 1960s, he would have been a candidate for electroshock; in the 1980s, he would have been inscribed with anxiety or stress and prescribed anxiolytics and tranquillizers, and in the 1990s, inscribed as depressed, he may have been given electroshock when the anti-depressants failed.[12]

Many novels feature protagonists who are mad, inscribed or incarcerated within psychiatric institutions. All lend themselves to interpretation from film or television directors and producers (for example, David Mercer's 1962 TV play, *A Suitable Case for Treatment*. See also Marketing and movies).

Chekhov's novella *Ward No. 6* was written in 1892.[13] Szasz describes it as 'a powerful attack on the entire system of psychiatric incarceration.' For Szasz, 'Chekhov, himself a physician, knew whereof he spoke.'[14]

Pat Barker uses the contrast between Yealland's violent 'treatment' of shell shock to Rivers' kindlier approach to her character Billy Prior in *Resurrection*.[15] Devastated by his experiences in the trenches of the First World War, Prior returns to England to be treated by W.R. Rivers, a psychiatrist and one of the founders of the *British Psychological Society*. Yealland, also a psychiatrist, claimed to have overcome mutism in shell-shocked soldiers by giving electric shocks to the back of the throat; if the patient screamed, he was by definition cured.

Rivers preferred gently chatting to people. For 'Billy' and thousands of others the outcome was much the same; they returned (as did the poet Wilfred Owen) to almost certain death in the trenches. Rivers was in the position of being paid as an analyst and psychiatrist to send young men back to the front. It was something he almost achieved with the poet and writer Siegfried Sassoon, perhaps one inspiration for Barker's novel. As Szasz has noted (see above) the convergence of psychoanalysis and psychiatry was equally convenient for authorities in World War Two.

French physician-and-novelist Laurent Seksik's historical novel examines the tragic life of Eduard Einstein, son of Albert and his first wife, Mileva Maric. Seksik relates the encounter between Manfred Sakel (see Inscription and Insulin coma) and Mileva and the way Eduard had been subjected to insulin coma after his inscription with schizophrenia.[16]

Caleb Carr's *The Alienist* (now also a Netflix series) manages to be sceptical of the mysterious knowledge of psy experts while maintaining the myth they know more about human motivation than ordinary folk. To all intents and purposes it is a murder mystery telling the tale of a nineteenth century New York Police Commissioner who is seduced by the magic of psy expertise and, secretly, enlists the help of an alienist to catch a serial killer.[17]

Elaine Showalter explores themes and gender stereotypes with particular reference to the psychiatrist/guru Ronnie Laing and the work of Doris Lessing. Lessing claimed an affinity with madness via her contact with various therapists and psychiatrists saying: 'I have always been close to crazy people.' [18]

For Showalter, Laing, Lessing and Clancy Segal (author of *Zone of the Interior*, a comic novel about his time acting – under Laing's direction – as a schizophrenic), 'formed a circle of almost incestuous mutual influence.' With Laing, David Cooper, Aaron Esterson and Sid Briskin, Segal formed the Philadelphia Association and its first therapeutic community Kingsley Hall, where LSD and confrontational group meetings were meant to reveal the enlightenment underlying madness and rage (see Research and Robeson).

Showalter suggests that Lessing's 1960s' fiction parallels the change in Laing's view of madness from a reaction to competing familial demands to a form of rebellion against an insane society. Using schizophrenia as a metaphor for female consciousness, the heroine of 1962 novel *The Golden Notebook,* struggles to reconcile her Marxism, maternal feelings, sexuality and literary ambition.

By the time of *The Four-Gated City,* Lessing is railing against psychiatry (the heroine is inscribed, electro-shocked and given insulin coma); the novel is partly about the societal position of woman as represented by a male-dominated Psy complex. Showalter claims that, with the publication in 1972 of *Briefing for a Descent into Hell,* Lessing has made the Laingian circle complete. Here madness, as represented again by schizophrenia, is 'a voyage into a more authentic world.'[19] The protagonist is no longer female and, after 'treatment' with a cocktail of psycho-active drugs and electroshock, re-enters the world a sad facsimile of his former self.

Opposition
and Oprah Winfrey

There have been campaigns against most psy treatments for over a century and a half – from the Alleged Lunatics' Friend Society of the mid-nineteenth century to Witness today.[1] There are several websites devoted to critiquing electroshock.[2] Facebook and related media are a source of information from survivors.[3] Campaigners aim to make the practice more *visible*.

Thomas Szasz rightly says that campaigns and electroshock-opposition, though understandable, miss the target. If psychiatry doesn't 'cure' real illness then debates about which treatment is bad or best miss the point.[4] A significant problem with opposition movements is the promotion of 'alternative treatments' – psychotherapy rather than drugs, and so on – but if distress is integral to the human condition, it doesn't need inscription and therapeutics. Amelioration via comfort, massage, friendship, gin, whatever, should perhaps be preferred to facing the machinations of psy.

In the late 1990s my Shropshire neighbour's 40-year-old son was killed in a climbing accident. By now almost 80, the neighbour was overwhelmed with grief. A few days after the accident his wife called to say he had been admitted to the local psychiatric hospital and the consultant psychiatrist was considering electroshock. Though employed by the same hospital as a clinical psychologist, I visited in my capacity as a friend. I reminded my neighbour that he was a voluntary patient and couldn't be compelled to undergo treatment.

He asked me to sit in on his case conference as an advocate. I was asked into the tail end of a discussion about a previous patient, just at the point where a nurse was telling the consultant that the patient's spirits 'seemed to be lifting a bit' after her second bout of shock treatment (see Precision and Mervyn Peake). The consultant nodded sagely and recommended that the 'course of treatment' (four more sessions) should be completed.

During his own case conference, my neighbour refused further shocks and, supported by his wife, was discharged the following day. That day I was called to the Director of Mental Health's office and informed I had been banned from the ward.

Meanwhile, the bus from Ellesmere to Shrewsbury continues to be a source of inspiration. The 501 is a community of fellow travellers who chat on four or five days each week with only a vague idea of where each other actually lives – imagine a train journey where you find yourself saying all sorts to a stranger or listening in as a fellow passenger makes long calls on a mobile phone. I have sold and given away copies of CDs on the 501, have written 000s of words for various projects and I am now writing this to email to myself later.

Ten years ago I met a couple who would sit chatting to each other or fellow passengers. Two years back, I noticed that the man was often asleep. He once overheard my remark to his partner that I admired his ability to doze and he responded with anger. A year later I discovered he was in hospital with an undiagnosed problem. During a long conversation with his partner, I was told he had been in and out of the local psychiatric unit for twelve months. He has been inscribed with depression and received electroshock as well as Lithium. He is 80, shows no sign of change and his partner is uncertain whether or not to suggest to the consultant that he returns home for her to care for him. Her diagnosis? 'Grumpiness.'

She is confused about the inability of 'well qualified' consultants to get to the root of his problem – if problem it is; grumpiness isn't yet a disorder and she wonders aloud if 'intolerance of grumpiness' is her problem. Her solution – to care for him as if she has marriage vows to fulfil – will be as challenging as any partnership on the ropes.

Unlike many others, and partly through shame, she won't be helped by other carers and activists. As yet, she has not identified with any particular group – activist or otherwise. Perhaps this is for the best as groups, particularly strident protest lobbies, tend to be absorbed by the system of governance against which they are speaking out.

Social psychologists have classified the ways people may be grouped in terms of referent and nominal groups. Broadly, a referent group has importance for group members in terms of shared identity while a nominal group has demographic and potentially environmental significance. For example, a feminist collective will identify with the shared political agenda of citizen rights. If the group is predominantly women, they may share nominal similarities that can be ignored or exploited by other agendas. For example, advertisers will target a perceived demographic as potential mothers, wage-earners, consumers with the power to purchase products aimed at 'women', and so on.

Psy has similar strands. Nominal identities (over 60, male, female, (un)employed, 'adolescents' and so on) may be noted in anonymised research publication. For those receiving psy interventions there are numerous self-inscribed identities available. As evidenced by Facebook and other social media, many groups identify with formal inscription of bipolar, ADD, etc. For the psychiatric protest movement, self-inscription includes: survivors, patients, recipients, people, experts by experience, consumers, consumed, clients, activists, citizens and users. The survivor movement prefers the term 'survivor' due to the 'inhumane, hurtful, degrading and judgemental ...' nature of psy.[5]

One of the most passionate critics of electroshock, Leonard Roy Frank (see Evidence and Electrocution and Inscription and Insulin coma) can be seen speaking out about psychiatry on Youtube.[6] Frank is not alone. Activist survivors include Viv Lindow (see History and Hemingway) who went on from her experiences of electroshock to complete a doctorate in psychology to add the weight of legitimate authority to her voice. She then began to protest about the entire system, eventually recommending leaving the system at the earliest opportunity in order to join or set up survivor led alternatives. The disadvantage to this move is in staying connected to a survivor identity and expending energies for those with similar identities thus risking ongoing involvement with formal psychiatry, even if only acting as a consultant to the system.

It is a form of engagement common to those who protest against numerous elements of post-industrialism – road building, aeroplane travel, militarism, and so on. The surge in new medical praxis ensures a proportion of patients harmed by new interventions or 'rogue' physicians. These too become the focus of protest, but the lives protestors previously spent getting on with day to day living are now exclusively dedicated to the exhausting work of protest and campaigning.

Lindow stresses that although she values many 'alternative' (actually age-old) therapies, survivor-led resources act as alternatives to the warehousing, incarceration and physical invasion (see Death-making and David Reville) commonly found in formal psy praxis. Inspired by the work of Judi Chamberlain (specifically by her best-selling On Our Own[7]) Lindow promoted schemes in Sweden, London, Sheffield and Oxford in the UK, North America and Japan.

Termed either survivor- or user-controlled the projects range from providing friendship and contact through day clubs to employment schemes and places of refuge or simply places to live without the stigma attached to 'homelessness.'[8] Szasz is one of many authors to point out that the provision of somewhere to live has been the main function of so-called asylums since the establishment of the Bethlehem Royal Hospital or Bedlam (see Precision and Mervyn Peake).

Peter Lehmann has also carried his protest to activities beyond formal psy. As a survivor, he is now a publisher and founder of the European Network of Users and Survivors of Psychiatry (ENUSP). He was also the webmaster of the ENUSP website. The site includes articles, links, commentaries and information generated by survivors on the various iatrogenic effects of psy interventions.

The information appears in over 50 languages. The translations are provided by survivor activists around the world: one of my own contributions appeared in Japanese, Arabic and Finnish within days of it being posted. Many professionally run journals would be expected to take months to respond at all, without the translation.[9]

Lehmann was also instrumental in the foundation of the Berlin Runaway House. A self-help group for survivors, the Association for Protection against Psychiatric Violence (Verein zum Schutz vor Psychiatrischer Gewalt e.V.) was founded in 1989 as a mixed group of survivors and other activists. In 1990, a private donor bought the villa in north Berlin that became the Runaway House. After a further six years of negotiation with government agencies, a day-rate remuneration for people's stay in the house was agreed using §72 BSHG (Bundessozialhilfegesetz: Federal Social Welfare Law 'Help in special social difficulties').

As a consequence, potential residents were

restricted to psy survivors who were homeless or in danger of losing their homes.[10]

Oprah Winfrey

Carrie Fisher was inscribed as manic depressive and then bi-polar. Addicted to alcohol in the 1980s, she wrote her first novel, *Postcards from the Edge*. Soon after her death from a heart attack, feminist culture writer Anne Thériault posted a tweetstorm, a series of thoughts about how people celebrate Fisher as Princess Leia, but for her the real hero is General Organa — 'the older, tougher, franker version of the character seen in *The Force Awakens*.' Fisher's ashes were placed in a giant Prozac pill, a favourite possession.

In February 2011, Fisher revealed live on television to Oprah Winfrey that she had 'maintenance' electroshock every six weeks. Winfrey's surprise was shared by millions and a storm of activity on the Web ensued. Some myths about electroshock were repeated and other commentators took the opportunity to promote other interventions.

Liz Lockhart, for example, says in *Mental Healthy*:

'ECT uses bursts of electricity in the brain to produce a mild seizure. It is not known with certainty why this works although specialists believe it releases neurotransmitters in the brain and stimulates underactive parts of the brain.'[11]

As noted in Research and Robeson, there has actually been agreement for many years that it is the electric charge rather than the convulsion that is of most importance.

In populist journalistic style, Tim Jarvis at Oprah.com uses the headline 'Breakthroughs for Depression are on their way.' Again, he promotes the seizure and effectiveness myths suggesting:

'To date, electroconvulsive therapy (ECT) ... is widely acknowledged as the most effective weapon for treatment-resistant depression in a psychiatrist's arsenal, and often the last resort.'[12]

Precision
and Mervyn Peake

Narratives within psy are rarely precise. A shared language may give the appearance of mutuality but different words at different times mean different things to different people. Stories told and re-told enter the discourse and become mythic; as the adage says: 'Nostalgia is happy memories of something that didn't happen.'

Myths are reified within any historical writing. The history of psy carries myths illustrative of arguments for and against psy praxis. This is due to a failure by researchers to return to original sources, the challenge posed by understanding what previous generations may have meant by popular psychiatric inscriptions (some, for example, carus simply disappeared from the lexicon; others, for example schizophrenia changed over time and across countries. See History and Hemingway and Inscription and Insulin coma) and, in part, by the desire of certain writers to castigate previous psy theoreticians and practitioners as villains and fools or promote them as heroic and prescient.

An example is provided in the posthumous celebration of Pinel, acclaimed for humanizing French psychiatry at the end of the eighteenth century by, quite literally, releasing the female inmates from their shackles at the Salpêtrière asylum. The famous illustration used in numerous history texts is accompanied by the date 1792. In fact Pinel's assistant Pussin unshackled the maniacs in 1797 – two years after Pinel left.[1]

Similarly (as noted in Zealotry and Zelda Fitzgerald) Egas Moniz is frequently credited with being the psychiatrist responsible for the first lobotomies and was awarded the Nobel Prize in 1949. In 1890, however, in an attempt to alter the behaviour of six severely agitated patients, Gottlieb Burckhardt, superintendent of a privately run psychiatric clinic at Marin in the Swiss Canton of Neuchâtel, drilled holes in their heads and extracted sections of the frontal lobes; two patients died. Moniz was, in any case, a neurologist and the operations were performed by his assistant, Lima.

Julius von Wagner-Jauregg has been the only psychiatrist to receive the Nobel Prize – in 1927. Over the previous decade he had injected patients with malaria as a cure (fever therapy) for shell-shock and general paresis. It was introduced into the US in 1922; over the next twenty years the practice all but disappeared except for treating cases of general paresis.

Myths have flourished in relation to psy institutions as well as regimes and individuals. For example, although the York Retreat is frequently put forward as the first asylum to practice moral therapy, its founder, Tuke, simply systematized an already common approach. The approach fitted the disciplinary nature of Quakerism thus adding to the myth. Foucault analysed the regime as one which rendered inmates their own gaolers controlled by guilt and shame rather than shackles. Anne Digby, however, has shown that, although the Retreat used severe restraint less than was common at the time, in the first fifty years of its establishment a pharmacopeia including opium, Laudanum and morphia was employed.[2]

In similar vein 'Bedlam' has become a shorthand for wild and uncontrolled conduct in noisy, untidy and unhygienic places. The term is based on the supposed chaos that ruled at the original Bedlam (the Bethlehem Royal Hospital in South London) necessitating the caging of deranged lunatics. Patricia Allderidge notes the regular appearance of Bedlam in psychiatric histories as a kind of symbol of the worst excesses of in-patient alienism but also remarks on the fact that only *two* histories of the hospital are based on original sources.

One of these, she tells us is the 'practically unreadable *Story of Bethlehem Hospital* by E.G. O'Donoghue, published in 1914.'[3]

Allderidge goes on to review evidence for chaining of inmates, the filth, lack of care and general mayhem in a place where, it is said, thousands of visitors paid to see mad folk. There is, perhaps, an overemphasis on the rules at Bethlehem in Allderidge's reading, rules which emphasized care of its pauper inmates. For contemporary staff it is common knowledge that rules and guidelines are ignored for the sake of pragmatism. Hence the discovery in spring 1814 of ten female patients chained by one arm or leg to the wall of a side room. All were naked except for an unfastenable blanket gown. More notorious was the discovery of

165

James Norris, 'confined in a dungeon, his body enclosed in a device of iron bars and chained to the trough where he lay.'[4]

Nonetheless, that same spring thirteen women were discovered in York Asylum in a cell twelve feet by seven feet ten inches '... and the deaths of 144 patients had been concealed.'[5]

Thus, although 'Bedlam' has achieved the status of an icon, it was not unique in its callous treatment of some inmates. The scandal at Bethlehem Royal eventually led to the establishment in 1828 of the Board of the Metropolitan Commissioners in Lunacy to carry out licencing and inspection of London's madhouses and whose remit was eventually – via the Lunacy Commission – extended to cover England and Wales.

Ironically, as a charity, Bethlem was excluded from the strictures of the 1845 Act. Further, 'madhouses' may imply large asylums but the licencing of private lodgings was a greater demand on the Commission's resources. Lodgings were licenced for only one patient but multiple occupancy was frequent. Visitors did come to Bethlehem Royal but in nothing like the numbers claimed and were certainly not charged a penny a time – records in the collection boxes reveal virtually no small coinage. Again, the myth is more important than the reality; 'Bedlam' serves as a benchmark against which modern 'more progressive' regimes can gauge their efforts.

Equally dramatic points can be made by historians of electroshock – either to contrast the 'barbaric' procedures of the past with enlightened more cautious contemporary approaches or by quoting selectively from original documents (as a volume like this is bound to do).

Valenstein and Shorter respectively give subtly different versions of Bini and Cerletti's first human experiment with electroshock (see History and Hemingway).[6] More recently, Shorter and Healy report in more detail covering both the first days of experimental electroshock (raising the voltage each time) and the outcome.

The majority of conflicting accounts cover only the first session with 'Enrico X' crying out: 'Not another one, it's deadly' (the preferred translation amongst activists). For Shorter and Healy – essentially pro-electroshock – the phrase instead is rendered: 'Attention! Another time is murderous.'

After the second shock, a week later, the patient/guinea pig Enrico X recovered but had no memory of what had occurred. Enrico had a total of 11 electroshocks and returned to work. A page further on the reader is informed that in March 1940, two years after the electroshock, Enrico X's wife wrote to Bini to say her husband was in the Mombello psychiatric hospital.[7]

This more nuanced account doesn't prevent the authors repeating the Pinel myth as: 'the celebrated loosening of the chains of the inmates of the Bicêtre Asylum in Paris by Philippe Pinel ...'[8] As noted above, it was at the Salpêtrière – a practice already introduced at the Chambéry by Daquin, the first asylum director to recommend moral therapy.

Precision is also absent in the prescription of all psy interventions – from electroshock to psychotherapy – and equally absent in their application. There is, for example, no research justifying any given number of counselling sessions recommended for a patient; the number is based on what the patient, insurer or state will pay and sometimes what the therapist wants to earn.

Patients in psychoanalysis frequently pay for sessions when the analyst is on vacation on the basis that it is a way of ensuring the analyst's ongoing fidelity yet no research can confirm the ideal length of the analyst's absence. Similarly, counselling clients may be offered contracts in multiples of six. A contract of six, twelve or eighteen one hour sessions may offer the illusion of precision but the basis for the number again reflects economic imperatives and no research exists comparing, say, nine 45 minute with thirty one 17 minute meetings. As ever, there is a touch of magic to the proffered session duration – 12 mirrors the number of apostles (the reason hospitals often had twelve-bedded wards), six the traditional number for a carton of eggs.

The historical and contemporary practice of psychopharmacological prescription is similarly imprecise. As noted in Research and Robson, medicine favours an empirical approach; dosages are increased or decreased and drugs changed until the desired effect is achieved. Sandison's experimentation with LSD and *Rauwolfa serpentinia benz* at Powick is the tip of a considerable iceberg (see Research and Robeson). *All* prescriptions of psycho-active agents are best guesses – or sometimes just guesses. Physicians use drugs not recommended for particular inscriptions or in excess of manufacturer guidelines and patients self-medicate in non-prescribed ways on a daily basis.

Non-sanctioned prescribing practices are seen to be controlled to a limited extent by professional, manufacturer and government guidelines or 'best practice' (see Law and Lou Reed). General practitioners and other psychotropic prescribers, however, rarely, if ever, do precise checks of a person's body-mass index or metabolic rate before prescription; again empiricism is the norm.

From its inception, there has been an empiricist approach to electroshock. Bini tried one burst of electricity with no success; Enrico X ended up with 11 sessions of different voltages (see above). Although a few of the more famous electroshock recipients referred to in this volume may have had the same number of shocks, the voltages and anaesthesia would have differed in every case depending on the preferred practice of the prescribing psychiatrist and the type of device used.

Precision will not be found in either the reports of 'successful' electroshock or its adverse effects. We are informed that people may have a 'generally improved mood' or, in many historic accounts were 'able to return to work.' Beneficial and adverse effects – especially those in recipient accounts – tend toward all or nothing reporting. Kitty Dukakis talked of her demons being banished after electroshock (see Kindness and Kitty

Dukakis). Other personal accounts suggest the recipient 'can't remember anything' from before the shock.

The type of adverse effects highlighted is also subject to the prevailing zeitgeist. In an interview for *The Psychiatric Times,* Jonathan Sadowsky, author of *Electroconvulsive Therapy in America: The Anatomy of a Medical Controversy* discusses three factors in the accounts of memory loss resulting from electroshock: [9]

> 'The problem of memory loss has been studied virtually since the inception of ECT – which is curious in itself if the therapy is as harmless as some of its strongest proponents claim. What struck me most about this history was how inconclusive it is. Some advocates are convinced permanent retrograde losses are rare, and some critics are convinced they are very common. But many researchers have stressed how elusive certainty has been.'

He adds that, from the recipients' perspective:

> '... complaints about memory loss seem to appear more in recent patient accounts than they do in earlier ones ...This may simply be an artefact of the growth of illness memoirs, making more evidence available. It could also reflect how awful some of the more serious adverse effects were before the use of anaesthesia and muscle relaxants became widespread.'

Finally, he touches on the issue of zeitgeist citing historian Laura Hirshbein. She proposed that the increase in accounts of memory loss might be related to an increasing emphasis on cognition in an information-based society.[10] Underlining the lack of precision in psy accounts, Sadowsky says: 'None of these hypotheses are easy to prove empirically. I do think the narrative evidence shows that permanent losses may be more common than some clinical manuals allow.'[11]

Attempts to make assessments of the impact of electroshock via psychometrics are hampered by the low reliability and lack of construct validity of psychometric tests though some precision has been achieved by researchers looking at the extent of brain damage suffered by recipients (see Evidence and Electrocution).

As psy maintains the privileging of the brain in its view of madness and distress, so it continues to attempt physically hazardous 'treatments.' Mid-nineteenth century alienists identified the overwhelming complexity of the brain and the impossibility of aligning conduct to specific cerebral areas (see History and Hemingway and Inscription and Insulin coma). Their reluctance was in part because metaphoric constructs such as love or schizophrenia belong in dictionaries not neurons.

Contemporary researchers and psy professionals seem untouched by their forebears' caution. As noted in Zealotry and Zelda Fitzgerald, Repetitive Transcranial Magnetic Stimulation is gaining a fan-base. The conclusions from a recent trial are an example of the lack of precision common to psy writings:

> 'rTMS treatment for MDD targets the prefrontal
> cortex ... cells in this area connect to networks that
> project throughout the brain, and rTMS has both
> enhancing and inhibiting effects on distant brain
> regions. The full extent of these hubs and networks
> are *poorly understood*, but it *seems* clear that
> modulating the activity of the prefrontal cortex
> releases neurotransmitters deep in the ancient
> structures of the midbrain, in particular the caudate
> nucleus. In turn, *these structures regulate our basic
> motivations and emotions.* So by indirectly
> stimulating these regions, rTMS *seems* to correct the
> low mood and listlessness of MDD in *some* people.'[12]
> (my emphasis)

A generous reading of the above would be that
words like 'seems' and 'some' reflect scientific caution
and as a rhetorical device the words add rather than
detract from the perceived expertise of the writers. A
less generous reading would be that the researchers are
guessing as evidenced by the couplet 'poorly
understood.' And yet, they go on to claim: '... these
structures regulate our basic motivations and
emotions.' This mixture of guess-work and strongly
worded statements can render readers puzzled.

An article by psychologist Nick Davis concerning
rTMS. makes clear the guess-work involved in these
procedures:

'The number of parameters involved in rTMS, such as the number of pulses to deliver, or the intensity of each pulse, makes it difficult to specify precisely the dose required for a patient. Precision is also a problem in locating the exact target in the prefrontal cortex for stimulation – each person's brain folds in its own way, and missing the DLPFC even by a centimetre can mean the difference between a person being a 'responder' or a 'non-responder', in the stark language of psychiatry. Moreover, the physical sensation of rTMS, which can feel like a woodpecker tapping the head, makes it difficult to create a placebo condition for use in clinical trials.'[13]

Precision is bound to be lacking in inscription as diagnoses have neither validity nor reliability. The act of diagnosis is better regarded as conduct that validates the diagnostician as expert. That expertise has been questioned since psychiatry's inception. Lord Shaftesbury, who had witnessed scenes of manacles and squalor in asylums since his involvement in the 1828 Commission, was a constant thorn in the side of psychiatrists and, '... stated on several occasions that a layman could give as good an opinion on the existence of insanity as a doctor.'[14.] His position was played out in French courts during the second half of the nineteenth century as alienists battled to prove their insights superior to lay interpretations of madness; in effect the experts claimed to be able to 'see into' the minds of criminals and detect insanity; the question of morbidity versus morality.[15]

Shaftesbury's critique still resonates. Why is it, asks David Stein, that John Hinckley who shot President Reagan was found not guilty by reason of insanity but Jeffrey Dahmer, cannibal and serial killer, was found guilty?[16]

The overall lack of precision in psy is summarized by US lawyer James Kelley:

'Patients and their families need to know that psychiatry is an uncertain branch of medicine, that well-qualified psychiatrists frequently disagree, that they deal more in judgement calls than in answers, and that the risk of a bad outcome is sometimes high.' [17]

Mervyn Peake

Teenage years are a good time to more or less disappear into Mervyn Peake's *Gormenghast*. Steerpike is powerfully alluring, Fuchsia is growing into an independent woman and obscure, unattainable object of desire while Titus seems like he might turn out to be just another rich kid.

I read the trilogy in the wrong order; *Titus Groan* second and *Titus Alone* a couple of years later. *Titus Alone* is both prescient and deeply strange, a gothic world with flying *cars*.

Peake was born the son of a medical missionary in China, in 1911. By the time of his conscription in 1939 he was an established artist and author. Between 1943 and 1948, he finished *Titus Groan* and *Gormenghast* and illustrated Lewis Carroll's *Hunting of the Snark* and *Alice in Wonderland,* Samuel Taylor Coleridge's *The Rime of the Ancient Mariner,* and Robert Louis Stevenson's *Strange Case of Dr Jekyll and Mr Hyde,* as well as producing countless poems, drawings, and paintings.

For ten pounds, he designed the logo for Pan Books. His book of nonsense poems, *Rhymes Without Reason,* was published in 1944. In 1945, the *Picture Post* commissioned Peake to visit France and Germany for the magazine. He was among the first British civilians to witness the remaining prisoners in Belsen; too sick to be moved, they were dying. In 1946, the family moved to Sark, inspiration for the wonderful *Mr Pye.* *Gormenghast* was published in 1950, *Mr Pye* in 1953.

Increasingly erratic, by 1957 Peake was hospitalized with the early signs of dementia. He was given electroshock and over the next few years he gradually lost the ability to draw steadily and quickly, although he still managed to produce some drawings with the help of his wife. *Titus Alone* was published in 1959. Among his last completed works were the illustrations for Balzac's *Droll Stories* (1961).

Peake's health subsequently declined and he died on 17 November 1968 at a care home run by his brother-in-law, at Burcot, near Oxford. His death was the result of dementia with Lewy bodies.[18]

Written some time during the Second World War and published posthumously, *The Threads Remain* is Peake's attempt to 'classify his loves' because of his 'Disorganized desire to live.' It ends:

'So now I know myself and I
Can start my life anew,
Half magical, half tragical
And half an hour, or two'[19]

Queerness

Queerness is a term encapsulating Lesbian, Gay, Bisexual, Transgender, Intersex and Queer (LGBTIQ). Context determines the label used with the only noticeable addition being homosexuality (a word first used by Kertbeny in the 1860s), as this was the term adopted in the pathologising of sexual identity.

The *standard cross-cultural sample* is a sample of 186 cultures used by scholars engaged in cross-cultural studies. In 1976, Broude and Greene compared attitudes towards and frequency of homosexuality in the ethnographic studies available in the standard cross-cultural sample. They found that out of 42 communities: homosexuality was accepted or ignored in nine; five communities had no concept of homosexuality; 11 considered it undesirable but did not set punishments; and 17 strongly disapproved and punished. Of 70 communities, homosexuality was reported to be absent or rare in frequency in 41, and present or not uncommon in 29.[1]

Male homosexuality in China, known as the *pleasures of the bitten peach, the cut sleeve,* or *the southern custom,* has been recorded since 600 BCE. These euphemistic terms were used to describe behaviour, not identity. Homosexuality in Japan (shudo or nanshoku) has been documented for over a millennium. Male homosexuality was normal in ancient Greece (Plato eventually changed his view that love between men was superior to heterosexual love).

In ancient Rome, the young male body remained a focus of male sexual attention, but relationships were between older free men and slaves or freed youths who took the receptive role in sex.

All the early Roman emperors with the exception of Claudius took male lovers. The Hellenophile emperor Hadrian is renowned for his relationship with Antinous. In 390 CE, Emperor Theodosius I made homosexuality a legally punishable offense for the passive partner and in 558 Justinian expanded the proscription to the active partner.

Among indigenous peoples of the Americas prior to European colonization, a number of nations had respected roles for 'Two-Spirited' people often believed to practice homosexual acts. While each indigenous culture has its own names for these individuals, a modern, pan-Indian term adopted by consensus is 'Two-Spirit'. Homosexual and transgender individuals were also common among other pre-conquest civilizations in Latin America, such as the Aztecs, Mayans, Quechuas, Moches, Zapotecs, and the Tupinambá of Brazil.

The Spanish conquerors discovered sodomy openly practiced among native peoples, and attempted to crush it out by subjecting the *berdaches* (as the Spanish called them) to penalties including public execution, burning and being torn to pieces by dogs.[2] Richard the Lionheart, Philip II Augustus, and William Rufus were engaged in same-sex relationships and Socrates, Lord Byron and Edward II, have been described as gay or bisexual; Foucault, however, regards this view an anachronistic introduction of a contemporary social construct of sexuality foreign to their times.[3]

Cultures influenced by the Abrahamic religions (principally Judaism, Islam and Christianity), the law and church established sodomy as a transgression against divine law or a crime against nature and deserving of the death penalty (Leviticus, 20:13). Indeed, in 1533, Henry VIII declared that sodomy be enshrined in English law as a criminal act – this represented a move from religious to secular conceptualisations of homosexuality.

This law, which was re-enacted in 1563, was the basis for all male homosexual convictions until 1885, when the Criminal Amendment Act (48 & 49 Vict. c.69) extended the legal sanction to any sexual contact between males. The Act also strengthened existing legislation against prostitution and made further provision for the protection of women and girls, and the suppression of brothels.

By contrast, Tulchin cites evidence for a form of male same-sex marriage in Medieval France. The legal category affrèrement (embrotherment) allowed two men to share living quarters, pool their resources, and effectively live as a married couple. The couple shared 'one bread, one wine, one purse.' Tulchin may have discovered the earliest form of same-sex marriage.[4]

The earliest extended defence of homosexuality in English, *Ancient and Modern Pederasty Investigated and Exemplified*, by Thomas Cannon, was published in 1749 and suppressed almost immediately. It includes the passage, 'Unnatural Desire is a Contradiction in

Terms; downright Nonsense. Desire is an amatory Impulse of the inmost human Parts.'[5] Around 1785, Jeremy Bentham wrote another defence finally published in 1978 in the *Journal of Homosexuality*. Despite these appeals, executions for sodomy continued in the Netherlands until 1803, and in England until 1835.

Between 1864 and 1880 Karl Heinrich Ulrichs published a series of twelve tracts, which he collectively titled *Research on the Riddle of Man-Manly Love*. In 1867, he became the first self-proclaimed homosexual person to speak out publicly in defence of homosexuality when he pleaded at the Congress of German Jurists in Munich for a resolution urging the repeal of anti-homosexual laws. *Sexual Inversion* by Havelock Ellis, first published in 1896, challenged theories that homosexuality was abnormal, as well as stereotypes, and insisted on the ubiquity of homosexuality and its association with intellectual and artistic achievement.

Although medical texts like these (written partly in Latin to obscure the sexual details) were not widely read by the general public, they did lead to the rise of Magnus Hirschfeld's Scientific Humanitarian Committee, which campaigned from 1897 to 1933 against anti-sodomy laws in Germany. In his final edition of *Sexual Inversion*, Havelock Ellis acknowledges Hirschfeld as the leading authority in the field after the publication of the latter's *Die Homosexualität*.[6]

Among many Middle Eastern Muslim cultures

egalitarian or age-structured homosexual practices were, and remain, widespread and thinly veiled. The prevailing pattern of same-sex relationships in the temperate and sub-tropical zone stretching from Northern India to the Western Sahara is one in which the relationships remain either gender-structured or age-structured or both.

In recent years, egalitarian relationships modelled on the Western pattern have become more frequent, though they remain rare. Same-sex intercourse officially carries the death penalty in several Muslim nations: Saudi Arabia, Iran, Mauritania, northern Nigeria, Sudan, and Yemen.

Today, governments in the Middle East often ignore, deny the existence of, or criminalize homosexuality. Iranian President Mahmoud Ahmadinejad, during his 2007 speech at Columbia University, asserted that there were no gay people in Iran.[7] Gay people live in Iran, however they are forced to keep their sexuality veiled from the hostile hierarchy, funded and encouraged by government legislation.

The few surviving poems of Sappho are the first European text to celebrate female to female love and desire. Havelock Ellis speculated that female 'inversion' was more common than in males but socially tolerated because men viewed it with 'amused condescension.'[8] His position directly contradicted that of William Acton, author of *Functions and Disorders of the Reproductive Organs* who '...regarded it as an insult to woman to consider her capable of sexual responses.'[9] Indeed, the Victorian wife submitted to sex and felt good *because* she didn't enjoy it – an inverted sado-masochism.

The ambivalence, fear and social unacceptability of same sex relations between men provided rich ground for alienists and psychiatrists expanding their claims to expertise. Homosexuality was pathologised for the first time by Ellis and Symons[8] when the term, along with paedophilia and transvestism, was added to a list of sexual deviancies identified in Krafft-Ebing's *Psychopathia Sexualis*.[10] This occurred in a context of perceived deviancy, sin and extreme stigma.

Oscar Wilde's disgrace, incarceration and eventual impoverished death in Paris, is a kind of testament to fin de siècle hypocrisy. In the first part of the twentieth century Queerness continued to be associated with criminality, sin and deviance. Those found guilty faced social exclusion and the choice of prison or treatment in the form of chemical castration. Wilde avoided castration though 20 years later Nijinsky (see Vested interest and Vaslav Nijinsky), who saw his own distress as a form of shell-shock, could not avoid insulin shock. His openly homosexual life-style would have added to Bleuler's conception that the dancer was disordered – in Bleuler's view schizophrenic.

Electroshock should be differentiated from electric shock treatment, historically administered as 'conversion therapy' for people who identified as Queer. Queers, predominantly men, either submitted to or were forced to have electric shocks delivered in relatively low frequent doses as behavioural conversion therapy or single high doses as electroshock.

Such approaches were by no means limited to psychiatrists. In 1961 Rachman, a psychologist based at the Institute of Psychiatry reported that he had:

'... utilized both photographs and imagination in the treatment of a man who was sexually aroused by women's buttocks and bloomers ... aversive conditioning sessions incorporated photographs of women in bloomers and imagined scenes of bloomers and of women with attractive buttocks. Electric shocks were applied to the fingers 10 to 15 times for each stimulus at each session. ...the patient said he no longer felt attracted by buttocks and disposed of his collection of pornographic photographs.'[12]

There are some similarities between electroshock and aversion therapy, as the former can be positioned as one type of the latter (see: Torture). Aversion therapy – rebranded positive punishment conditioning – when used to address sexuality is more commonly known as conversion therapy; therapy that seeks to convert the sexual preferences of the recipient. Whereas administering electric shocks to address sexual preferences was officially underpinned by the concepts of behavioural psychology, electroshock was not.

One factor in determining whether something is abnormal is supposedly its frequency in the general population, although Foucault would argue that normality is actually defined by default; declaring that certain conduct is 'abnormal' narrows the possibilities for conduct considered normal (see Governmentality and Gene Tierney). In the years preceding homosexuality's inclusion in the first Diagnostic and Statistical Manual of Mental Disorders (*DSM-I*), it was considered by official psychiatry to be relatively rare; statistically speaking, an outlier.[13]

The concept of 'outlier' is dependent on the notion that conduct is *visible* whereas homosexuality's criminal status ensured it was unknown how many people were bi- or homosexual. People continue to hide their sexual preferences within apparently heterosexual relationships and 'coming out' is heralded as a brave public act. Its so-called rarity was one of the arguments for homosexuality's inclusion in the *DSM-I*. Lou Reed's parents denied that his bi-sexuality had spurred them to arrange electroshock for him in Creedmore but, within the terms of *DSM-I*, Reed was homosexual (see Law and Lou Reed).

DSM-I listed homosexuality as one aspect of sexual deviancy of a sociopathic nature; other definitions within the category of deviancy included those for paedophilia and transvestism and may have perpetuated the myth that one must be linked with the other.

There is a resultant false conflation of homosexuality with sexual proclivity for children. In 1968, *DSM-II* continued to associate homosexuality with paedophilia and transvestism; it defined sexual deviancy in general as any sexual act not concerned with coitus with the opposite sex.[14] Despite his

Rabbinical family background it was not a position held by Freud.[15] Rather, Freud positioned male homosexuality as a manifestation of *diverted* sexuality as an element of the Oedipus Complex.[16] He also acknowledged bisexuality as an innate disposition.[17]

Pathologising Queerness as the diagnostic sub-category of homosexuality led to an influx of gay men, lesbians and transvestites to psychiatric hospitals. Some went 'willingly' though the general view of Queerness as something criminal, deviant or a disease impacted on decisions to seek treatment. One victim of conversion therapy described representation in the media: 'my entire emotional life was being written up in the papers as utter filth and perversity.'[18] Others reported that seeking support from family and general practitioners was met with moral judgements, discrimination and rejection.

In addition to electroshock and, in at least one documented case, leucotomy of a homosexual man, the use of electricity as a treatment was prevalent from the 1940s to the 1960s as a form of conversion therapy. Techniques involved administering electric shocks to the genitals or hands of homosexuals during the presentation of same-sex erotic stimuli. Conversion therapy using electric shocks finally fell out of favour due to a lack of efficacy, methodological flaws, poor follow-up data and questionable ethics.

Individuals who underwent treatment often left feeling shame, confusion and guilt about their sexual identities; some went on to commit suicide.[19]

Prevalence of specific treatments in psychiatric

asylums is not known because comprehensive records were not kept, though it is known that aversion therapies were peaking in the late 1960s.[20] Literature searches of the clinical evidence base provide scant information on the use of electroshock on people admitted to psychiatric units for treatment of their sexuality; accounts from nursing staff and patients, however, suggest uncontrolled and unethical practice of electroshock was rife. Overcrowded wards were placed under greater pressure due to the admission of Second World War veterans. As now, electroshock was given based on an individual psychiatrist's preference and with a poor evidence base.[21]

Studies by psychologists and sexologists were gaining traction in a social climate where direct action and progressive attitudes challenged the assumptions of psychiatry, refuting claims that homosexuality was rare or associated with various psychological factors.[22] The Stonewall riots in the USA, generally considered the catalyst for gay liberation in the West, galvanised activist groups. In 1970-1971, they disrupted the annual meeting of the American Psychiatric Association (APA), challenging the inclusion of homosexuality in the *DSM-II*.

In 1973, due to pressure from social activists (and, it might be speculated, the fact that a fair proportion of people on the DSM committee were secretly gay), the term 'homosexuality' was removed from the *DSM-II* (7th revision) list of sexual deviances.[23] Instead, the inscription of ego-dystonic homosexuality was introduced, essentially not liking being homosexual. It would, perhaps, be surprising if individuals inscribed in this way *liked* their sexual orientation given almost two millennia of persecution.

Research
and Robeson

The questions posed within psy research mimic the hypotheses of science though psy's research subjects, people, are in relationships with researchers and others that are transitory and non-replicable. A combination of the publishing imperative (for academic researchers), the promise of cultural (and financial) capital, curiosity and a poignant lack of reflexivity maintains research praxis in the face of nosological, methodological, philosophical and ethical challenges.

Research is the bed-rock of any discipline claiming to be a science. This is unfortunate for the so called human sciences. Clinical psychology, for example, has had a median research rate of zero since the Boulder Conference declared the arrival of the scientist-practitioner in 1949. The majority of psy professionals seem drawn by curiosity and concerns about humanity (themselves and other people) rather than a desire to perform experiments.

Once qualified, the majority of non-medical psy professionals get on with the business of trying to understand and help people using a technicalized battery of moral orthopaedics. For example, there are around 600 forms of psychotherapy[1] and major schools can be shown to dominate the zeitgeist during particular eras. A simplistic overview might suggest that the rise of psychoanalysis mirrored (and benefitted) the rise of advertising in the 1920s, remaining dominant until the rise of behaviourism (particularly in the UK) in the 1950s. The latter was matched by the importation of counselling from the USA and, by the time the baby-boomers of the 1960s arrived with money to spare, there was an eruption of therapies of 'self-discovery' and 'growth' rather than for specific forms of malaise.

For the majority of medically qualified professionals not working in the Academy experimentation is an unacknowledged daily event. As every individual's metabolism is unique prescribers can't know what a particular drug or combination of drugs will do to a patient. The picture becomes extremely complex if variables like physical fitness, body-mass, alcohol consumption, caffeine intake and other dietary factors are taken into account and would be impossible to gauge if environmental contingencies could be assessed.

The accepted approach in medicine is the empirical process: 'Try this. If it works, continue, if not, change the dose, add another drug or try a different one.'

Research in the Academy never reflects the complexity of real life; subjects are selected to approximate to a particular demographic – age, race, sex, and so on. Clearly, these can be wide parameters – 'age ranges' are used most often (as if a 20 year-old is similar to, say, a 25 year-old in the range 20-25), 'race' may be defined by self or other and 'sex' can be self-defined or determined via an experimenter estimate based on physicality. Within psy research the arbitrary nature of psy inscription (see Inscription and Insulin coma) renders categories such as 'depressed' or 'schizophrenic' equally arbitrary. Again, the experimenter is making a best guess (often using discredited psychometric tests[2]) at the appropriate inscription.

If an investigation aims to compare a treatment across experimental (inscribed) and 'normal' subjects, the definition of normal then begs a considerable question (see Normality and Novels). In fact, so-called normal subjects are rarely used in psychiatric research. Treatments and interventions are compared across inscribed groups but single interventions are not compared across inscribed and uninscribed subjects. If, for example, it was shown that a particular drug had the same effect on people whether or not they had been diagnosed with a so-called disorder, drug companies would not be able to market that drug for a particular inscription.

Over the first thirty years of the last century Havelock Ellis and Kurt Lewin, amongst others, published on the effects of mescaline but it was not until after the synthesis – in 1938 – of the ergot derivative Lysergic Acid Diethylamide (LSD) that medicine began to explore the potential clinical benefits of hallucinogens. By the early 1950s, experiments were being conducted at the Swiss Burghölzli clinic with people inscribed with schizophrenia and, in 1955, the 'LSD Block' was purpose built under the directorship of Ronald Sandison at Powick Hospital.

Sandison says: 'The process went some way towards fulfilling my dream of integrating traditional psychiatry with psychodynamics.'[3] His dream mirrors that of those who have tried to blend neurology with psychology, neuro-transmitters with diagnostic nosology or brain-biochemistry with psychotherapy. This is an endeavour bound to fail as metaphor cannot *ever* have a physical substrate; if two people cannot agree what 'depression' or 'love' are, how could they locate depression or love in the brain?

Joyce Martin, a Freudian analyst using psychotherapy with LSD at the Marlborough Day Hospital in London claimed to have 'cured' six patients of homosexuality.[4] She was not alone in her use of talk and acid; in the 1960s, the combination was used in Australia, Czechoslovakia, Denmark, Italy, and North and South America. As LSD became criminalized, so its use declined. But not before Ronnie Laing had become one of many psy professionals to 'drop in and drop out' alongside patients.[5]

In 1953, Samarin Banerjee brought, '...6 pounds weight of the roots of the shrub *Rauwolfa serpentinia benz.*' to Powick Hospital where he proceeded, with Ronald Sandison, to experiment on patients. Sandison's description of the way they prepared the root for their study is an object lesson in the way psychiatry substitutes scientism for science in its research:

'The British Drug Houses ground the roots up and put them in ten-grain cachets. The dose we settled on varied from 5 to 40 grains daily. I treated 108 patients suffering from a wide variety of psychiatric conditions...' Sandison records that the root had, '...been known for centuries for the relief of mania, and possibly schizophrenia.'

This is an example of a modern tendency to re-inscribe previous maladies. Schizophrenia, as a term, had only been used since 1908, 45 years before Sandison's use of the Rauwolfa root; whatever people before 1908 were suffering from, it was certainly not schizophrenia. He continues, '... it is of great value following ECT and insulin treatments. It can be used in conjunction with modified insulin treatments, alternating six weeks of each treatment, in schizophrenics in whom deep insulin treatment is contra-indicated...'[6] Paraphrasing Leonard Roy Frank (see Evidence and Electrocution) deep insulin treatment is now contra-indicated for *everyone*.

Although electroshock is claimed to be an evidence-based treatment, research in the field is on the decrease. A review of research articles on the practice between 1992 and 2001 revealed 117 articles, of which 10 per cent were randomised controlled trials. The majority of articles were North American (47%) and from the UK (14%).[7] *The Journal of ECT*, founded as *Convulsive Therapy* in 1985 by Max Fink, continues to publish the majority of studies (see Vested interest and Vaslav Nijinsky).

Two recent studies tackled the question of how electroshock affects patients' subjective memory worsening (SMW). Brus and colleagues examined Swedish registry data on SMW reported by 1,212 patients from a less than week before a course of electroshock to less than a week afterwards. A quarter said their memory had worsened, the majority women and younger recipients. Frequency and duration of stimulation, and electrode placement (unilateral, bilateral, or bitemporal) did not predict SMW.[7] In a prospective German study, 20 patients inscribed with 'treatment-resistant depression' completed neuro-cognitive measures before and at the end of their first course of 15 sessions of right unilateral shock and at one week and six months after completion of treatment. The authors suggest that: 'ECT produced substantial improvement in depression.'[8]

Claiming that: 'A large body of literature indicates that ECT is an effective and safe treatment option for elderly patients with major depression, even in very old-old age (more than 85 years)', Kerner and Prudic conducted a survey on research and practice in electroshock for older people. They suggest that: 'The efficacy of ECT in major depression is well established' and the antidepressant effects of shock are greater than any pharmacologic agent, including serotonin reuptake inhibitors.

They conclude that: 'For pharmacotherapy treatment-resistant major depression, 50 per cent or more can respond to ECT.'[9]

Sham electroshock involves taking patients through the entire procedure but, after anaesthesia, no electricity is passed through the electrodes. Given the likely adverse effects of electroshock, the conclusions of a review commissioned by the National Institute for

Health and Care Excellence (NICE) seem important. They say: 'In people with depression, real ECT is *probably* more effective than sham ECT but stimulus parameters have an important influence on efficacy; low dose unilateral ECT is no more effective than sham ECT. ECT is *probably* more effective than pharmacotherapy in the short term, but the evidence on which this assertion is based was of variable quality.'[10] (my emphasis)

Sham electroshock literature supports the conclusions that: real electroshock is no more effective than placebo, except during the period of time the shock is being administered. Even that difference is modest: 'A modest amount of cost is required for the overall cost-benefit of ECT to be negative; and, the effectiveness of ECT is overendorsed repeatedly...'[11]

Buchan and colleagues compared sham and real electroshock and followed patients up at four weeks and at six months. The study concluded that electroshock did have some beneficial effects, but only on those patients with physical retardation or delusions (a very small minority of those who are inscribed as depressed). In their words: 'real ECT does not appear to be effective in non-retarded, non-deluded patients' and any benefit was apparent at four weeks. At six months there was no difference between treatment and placebo groups.[12]

Ketamine (a N-methyl-D-aspartate [NMDA] glutamate receptor antagonist) has been used as an alternative stand-alone anaesthetic in electroshock for decades. Typically, it is a third-line or fourth-line choice (after methohexital or propofol), indicated when shock-induced seizures have become short or difficult to elicit. Risks include increased hypertension, tachycardia and occasional dissociative symptoms during the recovery period. Low-dose ketamine has multiple, complex effects on cognition and mood. Researchers began to study its use as adjunctive treatment in electroshock by cutting the induction anaesthetic with small doses of ketamine. It has been combined with various agents, including barbiturates and etomidate, but probably most commonly with propofol, a combination referred to in the anaesthesia literature as ketofol.[13]

Some anaesthetizing drugs including ketamine activate rather than suppress brain activity. It is categorized as a 'dissociative anaesthetic' and usually used on animals. At low doses, ketamine can trigger hallucinations. At higher doses, the excess brain activity leads to unconsciousness similar to the experience of seizure-induced unconsciousness following electro-shock. It can be injected, consumed in drinks, snorted, or added to joints or cigarettes. Sold on the streets as Super Acid, Jet or Cat Valium, it was placed on the list of controlled substances in the US in 1999.

Adverse effects include increased heart rate and blood pressure, nausea, vomiting, numbness, gloominess, amnesia, hallucinations and potentially fatal respiratory problems. Ketamine users also develop cravings for the drug. As it creates a detached, dreamlike state almost paralyzing the user it has been used as a 'date-rape' drug. Low doses of ketamine act quickly and are sometimes recommended for people inscribed with depression.[14]

Kellner's article in the *Lancet Psychiatry* describes this as 'an exciting therapeutic advance in the treatment of severe mood disorders ...' but adds: '... the early adoption and enthusiasm surrounding the clinical use of ketamine in treatment-resistant depression greatly exceed its empirical support' because 'ketamine's antidepressant activity is short lived' and there are, 'unknown risks for long-term cognitive side-effects, psychotic symptoms, and substance abuse.'

Rather than investigating the use of ketamine instead of electroshock, Kellner says that: 'combining the two therapies seemed a logical next step' while acknowledging that 'research on ketamine use in ECT has been starkly disappointing so far.' [15]

The research literature on the combined use of ketamine with electroshock comprises over 130 articles with few well designed studies (and none remarking on the invalidity of psychiatric diagnoses). A study by Anderson and colleagues of ketamine use with electroshock indicates that the pairing is no more useful than electroshock alone. The authors conclude: 'if a powerful augmenting or synergistic effect of ketamine in ECT existed, a strong signal would have emerged by now.'

Anderson's research indicates a 'greater than a small to moderate benefit... However, in our opinion, even a small-to-moderate benefit is worth pursuing. ECT remains the *gold standard* of antidepressant treatment and is essential for a large subgroup of patients who are seriously ill and resistant to treatment.'[16] (my emphasis) Not content with results to date, the Patient-Centered Outcomes Research Institute launched a funding campaign in 2015 for a study due to be completed in 2022. The study again compares electroshock with ketamine. The budget is $11,128,538.[17]

The practice of electroshock has long been acknowledged to be unsatisfactory, even by those who see a place for it. The UK *Royal College of Psychiatrists* has carried out three large-scale surveys but even the most recent one found that there were still serious deficits in the administration of electroshock, '...with only one third of clinics meeting *RCP* guidelines'. For example, staff were poorly trained and supervised, and some clinics used machines that did not allow a sufficiently wide range of current to be delivered, so that patients with a low seizure threshold, which can vary up to fortyfold between different people, were at risk of receiving too high a dosage.[18]

Despite these considerable difficulties – or perhaps because of them - research is now focused on cost-effectiveness and potential market competitors.[19] On a sheer treatment basis, repetitive transcranial magnetic stimulation (rTMS) is less expensive than electroshock. These prices vary by provider, but rTMS is typically in the range of $400-500 per session for a total cost of about $15,000. Electroshock is around $2,500 per session, $25,000 for ten sessions, plus the cost of a one week hospital stay in some cases.[20]

A review in 2005 set out to establish the clinical effectiveness and cost-effectiveness of electroshock for those inscribed with depression, schizophrenia, catatonia and mania. The researchers concluded that low-dose unilateral electroshock is no more effective than sham electroshock and: 'Shock is *probably* more effective than pharmacotherapy in the short term, but the evidence on which this assertion is based was of variable quality and inadequate doses of pharmacotherapy were used.'

'Limited' evidence, '... suggests that electroshock is more effective than repetitive transcranial magnetic stimulation (rTMS). Overall, gains in the efficacy of the intervention depending on the stimulus parameters of ECT are achieved only at the expense of an increased risk of cognitive side-effects. There is little evidence of the long-term efficacy of ECT. There was much less evidence regarding the efficacy of ECT in schizophrenia and mania, and no randomised evidence of the effectiveness of ECT in catatonia. The economic modelling results did not demonstrate that any of the scenarios had a clear economic benefit over the others.'[21]

A Spanish research group have provided a 'decision model' for comparing the cost effectiveness of electroshock and rTMS. The authors first contextualise the need for such a framework by reference to '... scarce healthcare resources' that require decision-makers to '... compare healthcare strategies, not only in terms of clinical effectiveness, but also in terms of their economic consequences.'

Understandably, the authors make no reference to Sartre's position that so-called decisions are retrospective justifications of actions. They also fail to remark on the possible unconscious factors in intervening in particular ways with particular patients (see Women).

They note that cost-effectiveness of electroshock compared to rTMS has been considered in previous published studies but with conflicting results. Researchers have found that rTMS alone offers a considerable economic benefit on healthcare and patient costs over electroshock alone, and that rTMS followed by electroshock was the most effective and least costly option. Another group found that rTMS was not cost-effective compared with shock; rTMS was found not to be as effective as shock and there were generally no differences on healthcare costs; informal care costs were higher with rTMS.

The Spanish group conducted an economic evaluation comparing electroshock with rTMS for patients inscribed as depressed who don't respond to pharmacological and psychological therapies. They compared: electroshock alone, rTMS alone and rTMS followed by electroshock when rTMS fails. Their analysis of six rTMS vs electroshock Randomized Control Trials (RCTs) considered the costs that would be incurred by the Spanish National Health Service.

Combining the differences in costs and in Quality Adjusted Life Years (QALYs) they found rTMS alone to be on average less effective and more expensive than electroshock alone.[22]

In the UK, Oxleas NHS Trust advertises an electro-shock service 'accredited as excellent by ECTAS, the

Royal College of Psychiatrists ECT Accreditation Service'. Based in Queen Mary's Hospital in Sidcup, the Woodlands unit offers local patients and out-of-borough patients 'who have funding in place' both electroshock and rTMS. The latter service was launched in January 2017 for patients inscribed with 'treatment resistant depression.' The advertisement claims: 'We have already seen some positive results in patients' and goes on to give contact numbers. It does not mention the Spanish research findings.

Acknowledgement that social factors are a major (some might suggest sole) determinant of the likelihood of being marked as depressed does not lead psy practitioners to suggest social intervention. The appeal to notions of interiority and individuality is exemplified in the 'American Indian and Alaska Native Women and Depression FACT SHEET', available on the National Alliance on Mental Illness website:

'Many minority women experience depression and stress brought on by persistent racism, gender bias, violence, poverty, large family size and social disadvantages.'

Suggested amelioration of the misery brought on by such circumstances involves only the *non-sequitor* of psy intervention: 'medications, psychotherapy and electroconvulsive therapy (ECT).'[23] This can be read as a further colonializing move; as in any colonised culture the language and mores of the invading culture soon overwhelm the existing customs. The – for some –

romanticised view of indigenous culture is one of spirituality and community. Disruption to that spirituality and sense of cohesion is met, by the invading culture, with further oppression in the form of psy techno-praxis. Thus, for indigenous (First People) Australians and Native Americans, rates of mental illness inscription and subsequent prescription of medications are in excess of the rates for other citizens.[24] In North America costs of private electroshock are so high that a predominantly poor community such as the indigenous people receive far *less* electroshock than their wealthier, white counterparts.

In Canada, a promotional leaflet from the *Canadian Psychiatric Association* reads: 'When used properly, ECT is a safe and effective treatment which should continue to be available as a therapeutic option for the treatment of mental disorders'[25] (see also Marketing and Movies). The leaflet simultaneously positions electroshock as an intervention that might be used *im*properly and reinforces the legitimacy (*pace* Szasz) of psychiatry as a branch of *bona fide* medicine through the trope of 'treatment.'

The hidden sub-text is further disguised by positioning life's struggles as 'disorders.'

All of these tropes are used in a promotional leaflet for cranial-electrotherapy-stimulation:

'Designed collaboratively by world-class engineers and doctors, the Fisher Wallace Stimulator® uses proprietary waveforms to gently stimulate the brain to produce serotonin and other neurochemicals responsible for healthy mood and sleep. Proven safe and effective in multiple published studies, the device is cleared by the FDA to treat depression, anxiety and insomnia.'[26]

A scientific conclusion from the scientistic research of psy would be forced to conclude: around two-thirds of inscribed people claim to benefit from anti-depressants some of the time and scores on tests such as the *Hamilton Rating Scale for Depression* (HRSD) are reduced. Electroshock research indicates that real electroshock is no better than sham electroshock. Six month follow up shows that any marginal gains for real electroshock dissipate although some people will have moderate to severe memory loss.

Ergo, if around a third of people taking anti-depressant medication show no signs of 'improvement' and electroshock, with or without ketamine, is no better than effectively doing nothing (sham electroshock), a third of inscribed people should be left alone. The problem for psy is in identifying which third this should be; General Practitioners and psy professionals tend to respond to the most demanding patients or relatives of patients and the 'gift relationship' ensures that they are likely to give something in return for the secret sorrows revealed by patients.[27] A prescription is bartered for banter.

Research has consistently shown that the majority of people go through at least one spell of about a year when they feel overwhelmed or at a loss – for women this may be in the first year of new motherhood when the desired 'bonding' cannot survive late nights, various physical changes for mother and baby and, if the new mother has a partner, a distancing rather than 'togetherness' in that relationship.

Some family therapists suggest that so called 'post-natal depression' is for many women actually a result of discovering their partner is having an affair on the basis of feeling excluded by the mother-infant 'bond'. This position is reinforced by advice manuals urging new mothers to 'make an effort' to include their partner – as if looking after a baby was not effortful enough.

As Szasz, amongst many others, has remarked relationship challenges are moral concerns hi-jacked by the psy professions as if they are illnesses.[28] It follows that were prescribers to adopt a research schedule of only prescribing to every third patient such practice would require people who regard themselves as healers to step back and wait. Acknowledging that life is a struggle but not intervening may not fulfil the desire of a General Practitioner or psy professional to be seen as helpful but, within the research parameters set out above, such an interaction would be entirely consistent with the evidence.

The cost-effectiveness of such a strategy would be extraordinary – billions are spent by the National Health Service and insurers around the world on drugs and billions more on state benefits. A third of those costs would be saved as prescriptions were not given and inscriptions of 'disability' were reduced. It is an approach unlikely to find favour with either pharmaceutical manufacturers or potential patients. As Rapley notes:

'Psychiatric drugs and, more recently, psychiatric disorders themselves have now become sought-after consumer products in their own right. In an historically unprecedented cultural turn there is now, courtesy of the promotional outlay on marketing to doctors and the popular cultural penetration of the APA and Big Pharma's direct to consumer (DTC) marketing, a shopping list of assorted 'mental disorders' that people quite literally *want* to have.'[29]

Ten of the most advertised drugs in the US are medications for psychiatric and neurologic 'disorders.' Bhanji and colleagues conclude: 'DTC advertisements increase both new diagnoses of a condition and the proportion of prescriptions specifically for the advertised drug.'[30]

A report by the Kaiser Foundation says: ' … nearly a third (30%) of adults say they have talked to their doctor about a drug they saw advertised, and 44 per cent of those who talked to their doctor received a prescription for the medication they asked about. This means that 13 per cent of Americans have received a specific prescription in response to seeing a drug ad.'[31]

As noted in Marketing and the Movies, this kind of promotion of a health/illness discourse ensures profits for drug companies, and benefits-in-kind (for example, a no-blame position) as well as financial benefits for patients. Some patients will achieve the desired 'oblivion.'[32] Others will gain no benefit or be harmed and return to the prescriber who, acting on the empirical principle, will change the dosage or drug. The same principle applies to electroshock. Writing for the UpToDate webpage, Charles Kellner says:

'People undergoing ECT need multiple treatments. The number needed to successfully treat severe depression can range from 4 to 20, but most people need a total of 6 to 12 treatments. The treatments are usually given three times a week.'[33]

Further profits will be made as drugs are prescribed to counter adverse effects and maintain the gift relationship. Any research attempted along the one-in-three process outlined above would meet considerable resistance.

Perhaps most importantly, where research uses psychometric test results to indicate change in the patient, as these tests only assess how the forms are completed rather than being indicative of real changes in mood, the most cost-efficient process for researchers would be to instruct patients how to give answers indicating positive changes. Patients will require no further potentially harmful interventions and researchers can still gain cultural capital and research grants from publication.

Paul Robeson
Paul Robeson was born in 1898. By the time of his death in 1976, he had been a law graduate, an American

football player, renowned singer and actor and an anti-imperialist who supported the Civil Rights Movement. In 1946, he founded the American Crusade against Lynching organization. He was active in the Council on African Affairs (CAA) and blacklisted during the McCarthy era.

During a party in his Moscow hotel room in March 1961, overwhelmed by fears that he was being watched, Robeson locked himself in his bedroom and cut his wrists. He stayed at the Barvikha Sanatorium until September 1961. Later that year in London, he became suicidal and panicked while passing the Soviet Embassy. His wife Eslanda organised his admission to the Priory clinic and consented to electroshock. For nearly two years at the Priory, he was given 54 electroshocks, insulin coma and high levels of Paraldehyde, Seconal, Meprobamate, Sodium Amytal, Parstelin, Largactil, Tryptizol, Pertofrane, Nardil, Marsalid, Nembutal, Phenobarbitone, Steladex, Carbritol, and Delatestryl. While at the Priory, Robeson was monitored by British MI5.

Robeson's son Paul Jr. believed that his father's fears stemmed from attempts by the CIA and MI5 to 'neutralize' his father. He said that three doctors treating Robeson in London and New York had been CIA contractors, and that his father's fears and hallucinations resulted from being subjected to mind depatterning under MKULTRA, a secret CIA programme.

As part of this programme, at the Allan Memorial Institute of McGill University, Montreal, the CIA was funding experiments on the use of intensive electroshock and drugs to wipe out memory. They also funded Hans Eysenck, a psychologist at the Maudsley Hospital where Robeson's psychiatrist Dr Brain Ackner, worked.[34]

The drug and electroshock regime finished in August 1963 when friends had Robeson transferred to the Buch Clinic in East Berlin. In December, that year he returned to the United States where, apart from a brief role in the Civil Rights Movement in 1965, he lived out his life in seclusion.

Sadism and
Spike Milligan

Psy fetishizes the individual; little understood processes like thinking are assumed to be internal and available to scrutiny. Other equally mysterious processes are positioned as arising in the cerebral cortex and amenable to alteration through moral orthopaedics (for example, psychotherapy), pharmacology and electroshock. These processes include mood, feelings and impulses to behave in particular ways.

Most of these processes are experienced unconsciously – we may be aware of an impulse to write, yell or stare at the stars, but we are rarely aware of how that impulse arises.

This is rich ground for those such as psychoanalysts who claim to be able to discern unconscious drives hidden to the analysand. It is frequently forgotten that Freud's theories did not arise in the context of working with inscribed psychiatric patients – though some, like Anna O, had been considered 'hysteric' by Breuer. Rather, Freud's theory of the unconscious arose with wealthy Viennese and was one that analysts see applicable to all of us.

If that is the case, interesting questions can be raised about the desire to subject people to electroshock

– both relatives and patients. Although Freud made it clear that one motivation for his work was money, financial gain and the search for cultural capital are not, usually, unconscious.

In asking what drives psychiatrists to electroshock others or relatives to give permission for electroshocking minors and parents (or grandparents), it is entirely possible to conjecture a variety of entirely conscious motivations (see Vested interest and Vaslav Nijinsky). Seen from an analytic perspective, however, these drives will match the unconscious drives and defences ascribed to patients. A competitive, young psychiatrist with an assumed history of (repressed) Oedipal desires towards his mother may – in analytic terms – feel sadistic rage towards older women patients who refuse his early, quite genuine, attempts to help. This rejection may be met by electroshock.

In similar vein, a psychiatrist driven by sadistic impulses to shock others may defend against these feelings through an intellectual defence – while never fully examining the contradictory evidence for electroshock's effectiveness or following patients up to see how they are doing. Such hypotheses may appear far-fetched but if, for some shock doctors, their own practice involves the use of psychoanalytic concepts, it behoves them to use such concepts in explicating their colleagues' and their own wish to shock others – or occasionally each other.[1]

Abse and Ewing published on this theme in 1956 and concluded that shock doctors expressed thinly veiled hatred and violence toward their patients and equate punishment with electroshock.[2]

It is worth noting that the impulse to protest about electroshock (or write books like this) can also be framed as a defence against the protestor's sadism – sadism that is now turned towards hated authority figures.

Make 'em laugh

Analysts are inclined to say that humour is a form of sadism; stand-up comics create tension by pillorying audience members, swearing or building up to unexpected *punch*-lines. If oral-sadism is, indeed, an externalized self-hatred, then humour – especially humour at the expense of others – becomes a way for a self-hating character to find relief. The Peters Cook and Sellers were inscribed with depression and Stephen Fry has gained a degree of notoriety in 'coming out' as bi-polar.

But who was the best of them all? Millions discovered the Goons in the 1950s. Sellers went on to find fame as an actor, Michael Bentine became a cult TV star and Harry Secombe a comedian, singer and host of *Songs of Praise* (and, as it happens, alongside Jeff Chandler, a pin-up for my mum). Terence Alan Milligan KBE called himself Spike after hearing Spike Jones and his City Slickers on the radio (in 1948 they were number one in the charts with *All I Want for Christmas is My Two Front Teeth* – and who can forget their rendition of *The Blue Danube*?).

For six years in the 1950s, Milligan wrote 130 scripts for the Goons, a process he described in a *London*

Evening Standard interview as, 'driving me mad. I had a nervous breakdown. It's like a roaring pain. The loudest pain you'll ever get.'[3]

He suffered his first breakdown during Series Three. Towards the end of 1952, he became convinced that he had to kill Sellers. Armed with a potato knife he tried to get into Sellers' neighbouring Highgate flat but walked through the plate-glass front door. He was hospitalised, heavily sedated for two weeks and spent almost two months recovering.

In 1959, Ken Russell made a short 35 mm film about and with him entitled *Portrait of a Goon*. He found himself so famous by the 1970s that a letter addressed Spike Milligan, London found its way to him. He was a trumpeter, poet, playwright and an actor famous for improvising lines on stage; through nightly re-writes he had transformed the 1964 production of *Oblomov* at London's Lyric Theatre. One of his last screen appearances was in the BBC dramatisation of *Gormenghast* (see Precision and Mervyn Peake).

He had a genius with the one-off unexpected comment. In *Puckoon,* the church-tower clock has stopped; for our narrator this means: 'It's right twice a day.' His war heptology is a masterpiece of affectionate memoir, wry humour and critique of the madness of war.

After the war, Milligan had at least ten breakdowns, some lasting a year. He was given electroshock several times before being prescribed Lithium and appointing himself patron of the Manic-Depression Fellowship. With psychiatrist Anthony Clare he published, in 1993,

The Survivor's Guide to Depression, though it's more a book by Clare with our Spike as a kind of case study.

The year the book appeared, Milligan was 74. He regarded his latest bout with misery inscribed as depression as brought on by his mother's death. In that same year, he said this about his most recent electroshock, six months before, 'When the Nazis did this it was seen as cruelty. I used to wake up and not know who I was and didn't care.'

He added he'd like a portable shock machine to put himself to sleep immediately when bored by people's conversations. He had no ongoing relationship with a psychiatrist and believed he had inherited his hypersensitivity. 'My mother was highly strung. I remember seeing my grandfather in a rage, striking a servant.'

He was overwhelmed after being shelled during the Second World War:

'My life was like an egg in a shell, just waiting for someone to crack me open and fry me. A bomb dropped right near my head. I got battle fatigue. The war fried me.'[4]

Torture

Already famous and garlanded on stage and screen, Laurence Olivier raised the bar with his performance as an ex-Nazi torturing Dustin Hoffman in *Marathon Man.* His chosen torture was drilling and extraction of teeth without anaesthetic.

Psy has direct affiliation with torture in the involvement of members of the *American Psychological Association* in CIA interrogations. In late 2014, it was revealed that a company founded by two former military psychologists and APA members who urged waterboarding and other coercive methods against suspects secretly imprisoned by the Central Intelligence Agency and Department of Defense, had been paid US$81 million for work with the agency's interrogation programme from 2005 until 2009.[1]

Ostensibly an example of disciplinary governmentality, the US government renders the information about the incident almost invisible by its comprehensiveness. The summary has 525 pages; the full report has 6,700.[2]

Psychology has a long history of torture renamed 'aversion therapy' – people are placed on 'punishment schedules' mirroring laboratory experiments with rats. More tangentially and symbolically, psychiatry employs methods that, to the lay public, resemble torture and for the recipient frequently have the same impact.

In 1986, I applied for a clinical psychology position

at Worcester State Hospital in Massachusetts. Approaching the main door by way of a very long driveway was like stepping back in time. The buildings were vast, the grounds extensive and, apart from a few ground staff who may well have been patients, the place seemed deserted – palatial with beautifully cut lawns under an azure New England sky, but empty.

At Worcester, Henry A. Cotton had been an assistant to doyen of American psychiatry Alfred Meyer in the mid-1890s. After studying with Kraepelin in Europe, Cotton returned to the US and was appointed superintendent of the Trenton State Hospital in New Jersey aged 31. Appalled by the extent of restraint practised at Trenton he freed 96 patients from their shackles, introduced nurse training and occupational therapy and began to systematically study his new charges.

Unfortunately for the latter, Cotton, along with countless psychiatrists before and after him *assumed* that the insane must have some form of cortical lesion (or, in the case of Pharma-sponsored psychiatrists, a 'biochemical imbalance'[3]).

In the absence of finding any lesions, Cotton pursued the empirical method and administered intracranial salvarsan for syphilitics and tried glandular extract with no success for a decade. In 1916, he became convinced that focal infection was the key to intractable mental disorder, a theory first proposed by English surgeon William Hunter in 1900. Cotton soon extracted all apparently infected teeth from 50 of his patients – with no discernible change in their conduct.

In 1917, he set up a dental surgery at Trenton and started to remove tonsils as well. His quest for the root 'bacteriological invasion' led to hundreds of operations and many publications and conference appearances. By 1921, he was suggesting that the treatment was saving the state over $70,000 per annum as patients were discharged to the community. It is not clear if the figure took into account the cost of antitoxins, laboratory analyses, X-rays and the operations themselves.[4]

Between 1919 and 1921, some 10,000 teeth were extracted; 90 per cent of the patients also had their tonsils enucleated. In the continuing absence of any effect on patients' behaviour, Cotton turned to other potential sites of infection: stomach, duodenum, small intestine, gall bladder, appendix and colon.[5] He set about dissecting, resecting and removing these organs – anyone with a history of constipation was particularly likely to be a candidate.

With the death of his specialist gastro-intestinal surgeon, Draper, Cotton started doing the operations himself. He estimated a post-operative mortality rate of 25 per cent and a lower success rate of bowel surgery for those inscribed as manic depressive. Suspecting that only partial removal of the bowel was the problem Cotton moved on to full colectomies, 78 per cent of them conducted with women. Eventually, following a less drastic procedure, the proportion of women rose to 84 per cent. Cervical removal was the next step.[6]

Families responded to Cotton's self-promotion. Between 1916 and 1921, the proportion of people prepared to pay for themselves or their children rose from 11 to 45 per cent. The New Jersey State Commissioner of Institutes and Agencies published a *Review of Reviews* essay on Trenton and Burdette Lewis opined that all previous hospitals were now out of date.[7]

Eventually, the bubble burst. Asked by Meyer to thoroughly research the outcomes of Cotton's surgery, Phyllis Greenacre found a 'cure' rate of no more than 40 per cent compared to Cotton's claims of 87 per cent. Worse, those who had received the more extreme surgery were unrecovered or dead. Her findings were quietly buried. After a lauded visit to Edinburgh, Cotton's procedures became less extreme until, in May 1933, he unexpectedly dropped dead.[8]

The film *Taken* dramatizes the raw application of electricity to a victim; although the electrodes are unceremoniously plunged into the victim's thighs, the principle – jolting charges of electric shock – is not so far from that justifying the application of powerful surges of electricity to the brain.

Users of electroshock are quick to dismiss analogies of shock with punishment or torture. The process can, however, be experienced as either. Torture frequently involves the victim being taken from a relatively 'safe' place to a room specifically used for physical assault. Touching a person's head can be experienced as threatening; the placement of electrodes on the head is both potentially alarming and – if the person has been shocked before – frightening. Knowing a shock session is due creates a degree of trepidation and, for those who don't want to be shocked, more fear. It is for these reasons that electroshock users have been careful to downplay the history and image of shock and the reason electroshock nurses have a specialist role – to calm and prepare the recipient (see Marketing and Movies).

A greater challenge to those who wish to portray electroshock as benign rather than harmful is the impossibility of removing ourselves from a given discourse. Potential recipients can't 'un-know' the images of *One Flew Over the Cuckoo's Nest* or further media revelations about Lou Reed or Hemingway's suicide. Myth or reality, these images and memories form part of our embodied context.

Salespeople, too, have a particular image, as do advertisements. Television commercials feature actors pretending to be delighted with products or exaggerated claims for products that the general public fully understand to be fiction. Even placing advertisements between television programmes or movies adds to this fictional context – whoever went to the movies expecting to see the truth?

In his exposition of critical realist social constructionism (CRST), John Cromby discusses how, for social constructionists, 'the world we experience and the people we find ourselves to be are first and foremost the product of social processes... It is primarily the societal reproduction and transformation of structures of meaning, morals and discursive practices that constitutes both relationships and subjectivity.' Language (as the carrier of categories and meanings) is thus central. Discourses, shaping what can be said and done, 'condition what is likely to be thought'. As discourses are the products of embodied beings in a material world, for CRST, 'our embodied practices run alongside our discursive practices, shaping and constraining them.'[9]

Watching Youtube clips promoting electroshock is an activity many people will thus experience in the same way they watch commercials. The subjective experience of watching an enthusiastic advocate of shock is contextualised by previous experience of TV salespeople. Viewers won't believe much of what they see because their embodied beliefs about harm and the clearly theatrical production render any 'information' redundant.

These presentations and psychiatrists recommending electroshock to voluntary patients can only employ language and logic as persuasion. As Cromby has said: 'This privileging of thoughts neglects the complexity of interaction between feelings, body and context in which people are situated.'[10] You can't change the ways people are likely to think and behave simply by talking to them and many people are likely to continue to fear electroshock and see it as torture or punishment whatever is said. Psy gets around this via compulsion (see Law and Lou Reed).

Medicare figures show the use of shock tripled in Victoria State in Australia in the private health sector in six years. In 2007–2008, for example, 18,000 treatments were conducted. In Victoria's private health system use increased from 1,944 treatments in 2001–2002 to 6,009 in 2007–2008. Of the 18,000 reported treatments, 12,000 were in the public health system. Of these 18,000, 6,197 were compulsory and nearly three times as many women had shock treatment compared with men. Increasing numbers of patients who had been forced to undergo shock contacted the Mental Health Legal Centre claiming they were tortured.[11]

The experience of psy recipients is only one part of the story. Electroshock has also been explicitly used as torture. On 28 September 2005, Mental Disability Rights International (MDRI) released details of human rights abuses perpetrated in Turkey against children and adults in the psy system. *Behind Closed Doors: Human Rights Abuses in the Psychiatric Facilities, Orphanages and Rehabilitation Centers of Turkey* describes the use of electroshock without anaesthesia on psychiatric patients aged from nine years old.

The investigators also found evidence of children dying from starvation, dehydration and lack of medical care in 'Residential Rehabilitation Centres'.

The report documents Turkey's violations of the European Convention for the Prevention of Torture (ECPT), the European Convention on Human Rights (ECHR), the UN Convention on the Rights of the Child (CRC) and other human rights and disability rights standards.[12]

It might be speculated that Viv Lindow's strategy for avoiding further electrocution is on a par with the reaction of victims of torture who will confess to anything under sufficient duress (see History and Hemingway). The tactic is not unknown to professionals: "Patients know that if they say they are not getting better, they will stay in hospital longer. They will probably be put on stronger medication ... They might be given ECT.'[13]

It has been claimed that psychiatrists described using electroshock to torture prisoners of the French during the 1954-62 Algerian War:

> 'There are, for instance, psychiatrists in Algiers, known to numerous prisoners, who have given electric shock treatments to the accused and have questioned them during the waking phase, which is characterized by a certain confusion, a relaxation of resistance, a disappearance of the person's defenses.'[14]

The US Central Intelligence Agency trained Moroccan security services in the early 1960s in the use of electroshock to torture prisoners during interrogations. In 1961, King Hassan II had asked the Agency to restructure and train his own security service. Doctors supervised a wide range of tortures of political detainees at 'a purpose-built detention center. ... [It] also had several Page-Russell electroshock machines, which were routinely used on prisoners. During the post-shock periods, Moroccan physicians questioned the detainees, seeking information about opponents to the king.'[15]

For psychiatric staff, torture is the last thing they consider when administering electroshock. The procedure is assisted by frequently kind-hearted psychiatric nurses who believe that 'Doctor knows best' despite having witnessed the effects of electrocution; few psychiatrists or psychiatric nurses will have seen a patient post-electroshock without disturbances in vision, balance or co-ordination. Many will have witnessed in survivors post-shock memory loss of over six months.

There can be echoes of the good-cop/bad-cop trope during the procedure. This is illustrated in the documentary *We're Not Mad, We're Angry* where a gently persuasive female nurse helps a middle-aged female patient onto the couch pre-treatment and off again post-treatment. She suggests the patient's headache and grogginess will soon pass. Adding to the sense of assault, the camera angle positions the viewer as the recipient.[16]

Politicians are not immune. In 1972, Senator Thomas Eagleton withdrew from the Vice Presidential candidature role with George McGovern due to media interest in electroshock he had been given between 1960 and 1966. The electroshock wasn't identified as torture by Eagleton but the stigma and potential trial by media wasn't to be overcome.

Unhappiness and
the unknown

The US Constitution may preserve the right to *seek* happiness, but no-one has a right to *be* happy. The desire to escape pain and fear has been with us a long time. More recently, perhaps, there is a growing desire to escape boredom in a techno-world so accelerated beyond our capacity to govern it that a few moments contemplation can seem an eternity.

Just as movie car chases must become faster and more dangerous, perhaps the perpetual white noise of an industrialized world's need for speed has increased such that an exhausted majority seek oblivion through alcohol and licit and illicit drugs.

Opium was used by lakeside dwellers in prehistoric times.[1] Therapeutically active ingredients were not extracted until the nineteenth century, some 400 years after the innovations of Paracelsus. Until then, sleeplessness and nervous restlessness were treated with opium in the plant form, a medicinal use first encouraged by Hippocrates in Greece, and Pliny and Galen in Rome. Mixed with water and alcohol, opium was marketed as Laudanum, 'enjoyed' by as many artists and poets as those with inscribed disorders.

Widespread use of the preparation led to the 1868 Pharmacy Act, though Laudanum was freely available in pharmacy shops at the end of the century. Morphine, cocaine and bromides, initially hailed as wonder drugs, followed a similar parabola, their medicinal use being tightly proscribed by 1900.

Barbiturates as anti-anxiety agents were first manufactured in 1904. By the 1930s they had replaced bromide and chloral hydrate on the grounds they were safer. The risks of barbiturate dependence were not acknowledged for another 20 years. After the popularity of their alternative, meprobamate (still marketed by Wyeth as Equanil), waned, the first of the benzodiazepines, Librium, was introduced in 1960. Followed by diazepam (Valium) in 1963, the two drugs rapidly came to dominate prescribing habits: 'Between 1965 and 1970 prescriptions for benzodiazepine tranquillisers in England and Wales rose by 110 per cent compared to a 19 per cent increase for all psychotropic drugs'.[2]

Over this five-year period, the number of prescriptions for the main benzodiazepines more than doubled – from less than 5 million to over 12 million.

Some noted figures have received electroshock to avoid either their own unhappiness or the ire and concern of their immediate family, amongst them authors Linda Andre, director of the Committee for Truth in Psychiatry, Janet Frame, Ernest Hemingway, Robert M. Persig and Sylvia Plath; actors Judy Garland, Vivien Leigh, Gene Tierney and Carrie Fisher; musicians Bud Powell, Vladimir Horowitz, David Helfgott, Michelle Shocked, Tammy Wynette, Townes van Zandt, Peter Green and Lou Reed.

Dick Cavett, the American television talk show host,

Yves Saint-Laurent and Edie Sedgwick were all recipients.3 Some of these appear in this volume; all were unhappy at some point in their lives. Some, like Hemingway claimed that electroshock killed his capacity to write (see History and Hemingway). Like Sylvia Plath, he subsequently killed himself though many commentators suggest that Plath's death could be ascribed to her circumstances.

Some, like Ted Chabasinski, an American attorney, went on to become psychiatric survivor activists. Chabasinski first received electroshock aged six (surely occasional unhappiness, like sudden bursts of joy is the normal state of most six year olds?). Being unhappy is not a criminal offence; on the other hand being happy is fleeting and, for the majority, a matter of happenstance. Being persistently unhappy is, however, alarming to friends and family of the miserable person. For Chabasinski, unhappiness led to psychiatric referral and recommendation for treatment – his concerned parents trusted doctors. Those parents of unhappy children who find themselves shipped across US state boundaries for electroshock (see Youngsters) may be as concerned and trusting as Chabasinski's.

Persistent unhappiness is concerning to the person and others. 'Persistent' is, however, a matter of perception. I was once referred a patient for psychotherapy to avoid the probability that she would be electroshocked. Inscribed 'Pathological grief' she had been widowed some three months before on the death of her husband of sixty years. Her psychiatrist thought that three months of misery was 'long enough.'

He clearly had no conception that, in many cultures, a year is an expected grieving period. In the multi-ethnic and multi-religious culture of England in the 1990s there was no prescribed period. Thus, it was his personal opinion that counted.

As in any psychiatric categorisation, elements such as unhappiness are always a matter of judgement; first by the patient (or, in the case of children, parents or teachers), then by family members and, finally by psy professionals. Current discourse means that in Western industrialised countries, the word depression is frequently substituted for 'unhappiness' and a slippery slope towards formal inscription begins.

We live in a world of celebration of the self or families and 'friends' on Facebook, supposedly joyous rituals like marriage, the birth of a new child to a 'happy couple' (particularly when that couple is famous or a member of the aristocracy), finding employment, 'succeeding' in getting a university place and so on. These events are meant to bring 'happiness' to ourselves and those around us. But, of course, a perusal of divorce, unemployment or debt statistics shows how Facebook posts and other celebrations are, like happiness itself, transitory. (No doubt, US readers will dismiss this as a view based on a rather gloomy European intellectual and philosophical tradition – they're right.)

One impact of the promotion of the pursuit of happiness is a mismatch between our feelings and what we are told we should feel; a married woman with a good career, university education and new baby simply shouldn't *be* unhappy. It can be a short step to inscription and entry into the psy system.

Although 'depression' is frequently taken as synonymous with unhappiness, this is a culture specific phenomenon. Marsella's cross-cultural surveys concluded: 'Many non-Western cultures do not even have a concept of depression that is conceptually equivalent to that held by Western mental health professionals.' And: "Depression' apparently assumes completely different meanings and consequences as a function of the culture in which it occurs.'[5]

People living in non-Western cultures may experience unhappiness, mourning, grief and loss but they do not conceptualise these experience under a rubric of 'depression' and referral to a mental health professional is unlikely, electroshock even less so.

On being unknown

We have lived in an age of celebrity for over a century. Now, celebrity status comes via social media, television, highly paid PR companies and Youtube. For many years in the early and mid-twentieth century it came via the radio and a burgeoning newspaper industry.

Until the laws concerning compulsory education, however, in the early part of the nineteenth century in Britain few people could read and many wouldn't have known who was on the throne or where London might be (Londoners may have not known of anywhere beyond a few miles from the city).

Although millions of cheaply printed 'chapbooks' were produced by presses in the larger cities of England

and Ireland from the seventeenth to nineteenth centuries, their subject matter was tales, songs, rhymes and lists of the meanings of dreams. Any remaining space was taken up by specialist areas such as astrology or love divination rather than 'news' about actors, writers or politicians. Sold wherever an outlet was available (market stalls, shops, fairs, and so on) they were eventually superseded by newspapers, magazines and more substantial printed books in the nineteenth century.

The cult of celebrity might be said to originate with Charles Dickens who read and performed to hundreds in specially hired halls. His first readings were for charity, beginning with two performances of *A Christmas Carol* in front of 2,000 working-class people in Birmingham. The author turned professional performer in 1858. Between December 1867 and April 1868, he earned over £19,000 (the equivalent of almost a million pounds today).

Dickens might be usefully compared with Shakespeare. There are few records of Shakespeare's existence other than a marriage certificate and some documents concerning his children. He appears to have been an actor and stage manager. The first folio to carry his name appeared in 1623, seven years after his death. By then the plays had been extemporized in performance, changed and re-written by the players. Unlike Christopher Marlowe, for whom there is a great deal more biographical material – at least after his move from Canterbury and, in part, because he was considered a spy – 'Shakespeare' is more a cipher. The works were produced by numerous uncredited actors. Historians have suggested alternative playwrights as the true author, including Marlowe himself. It was the cult of celebrity after Dickens that required a figure-head; a genius who had single-handedly produced the sonnets, *Lear*, *Titus Andronicus* and the rest.[6]

This volume promotes some of that celebrity culture. Many of the examples of people given electroshock found fame as actors, novelists or were already in the public eye. But that is to ignore the millions of unknown people who have been harmed or killed by electroshock.

Daily news bulletins may tell of the newest actor to 'come out' as depressed; many will be publicity releases stored by editors until so called mental health is popular currency and likely to sell the news channel or newspaper (itself designed to sell advertised products and services). These revelations are not news to the people themselves or to those around them. The opposite happens for ordinary folk. Rather like unreported civil wars in Africa, the everyday electroshock of thousands of people is not 'news.' They become a statistic – helpful in writing books like these – but a figure that reveals nothing about their struggles to survive psy. They are the unknown.

At this point David Boyle's *The Tyranny of Numbers* might be seen to have an apposite sub-title – *Why counting can't make us happy*.[7] Ordinary and unknown people are frequently harmed rather than made happy by electroshock. Making them statistics adds insult to injury.

The known and those who want to be known through self-publicity have some responsibility for the present state of psy and the public's subservience to its discourse; ultimately a self-defining discourse (see John Cromby's work in Torture). 'Coming out' for those in the media spotlight and industry is seen as 'brave.' 'Speaking out' for psy professionals might be seen as a career-ending move.[8]

Those who publicly self-identify with the latest mark bringing cultural capital can be careless in the promotion of both the notion of disorder and treatment. Columnists in the UK's *Daily Telegraph* are on something of a roller-coaster in their efforts to come out. In February 2018, journalist Judith Woods responded to a news story concerning the desirability of a 'million more Britons' being on anti-depressants (see Marketing and Movies). Her position is not that taking pills is bad but getting the 'right' medication is imperative. Her article is simply an advertisement couched in the rhetoric of a survivor.

Woods says she has 'suffered from depressive episodes from the age of 14...' and claims that depression is a 'chemical imbalance' (see Justification and Janet Frame).[9] Notwithstanding the disappearance of the chemical imbalance theory over the last decade, Woods does not address the lack of validity in psy inscription, perhaps understandably given the place of the psy lexicon in public discourse and possible peer pressure from colleagues amongst *Telegraph* staff who have come out.

Critically, she does not address the experience of

numerous unknown survivors and current recipients of psy - 'silencing.' A psy inscription tied to a 'chemical imbalance' can be used as a way of saying: 'This is not my/your fault' or it can discount a person's opinion as the person is now officially mad. The 'no fault' aspect removes the person's moral agency; discounting the person's opinions renders their statements invalid.

Journalists (and others) who use their inscribed identities to gain cultural or financial capital might address the paradox that, if their beliefs and conduct is regarded as insane, then beliefs about 'brain biochemical imbalances' are also insane. Rather than accept and promote such identities. They might draw links between injury, sexism, disablism, racism and the loss of status and citizenship brought about for the millions of unknown people similarly inscribed.

Vested interest
and Vaslav Nijinsky

Any human endeavour can be observed through the lens of vested interest. The history of electroshock can easily be positioned in this way. Despite an (accurate) image of the procedure as a brutal way to treat others, psychiatrists continue to use it and a significant proportion of patients continue to opt for it for themselves or family members.

Since its inception, remarkable energies have been expended by protesters and activists (both recipients and psy professionals) to speak out. Protest about its sometimes lethal effects takes the form of marches, sit-ins, DVDs, TV programmes, research articles, academic critique, Facebook and other social media (see: Opposition and Oprah Winfrey).

Asperger's, depression, schizophrenia, ADHD, like any psychiatric inscription, are now embedded in public consciousness and popular discourse. The claim that such labelling from schizophrenia to depression is indicative of a valid physical disorder (with a 'breakthrough' in verification and treatment just around the corner) continues to be made.

Any 'explanation' for the persistence of such claims is to be found in the profits of drug and test publishing companies, the cultural capital of researchers and psy professionals and the vested interests of self-inscribing patients. A (usually disguised) motivating factor in psychiatrists' promotion of physical interventions is to place the discipline within the bounds of 'real' medicine, that is, medicine that deals with physically verifiable illness in physical ways. This position is made clear in an editorial from the *American Journal of Psychiatry*:

'Since the mind is the organ expression of the activity of the brain, we can hope that some day we will achieve a complete understanding of all mental illnesses as both mind and brain diseases. And that psychiatry will still exist until the illnesses themselves cease to exist - as the medical specialty responsible for the study and treatment of mental illnesses.' [1]

Health professions are quick to distance themselves from the notion of vested interest. After all, what is a health profession other than an organization set up for the public good? The public sees through this smoke-screen. Similarly the management and consultancy ethos that swept through the UK's National Health Service in the 1990s deceived no-one. As a private in the army might say of a new officer: 'Not another fool to lead us...'

Sometimes the smoke screen disappears, though rarely in public. Sitting in a management meeting in the early years of this century, my boss whispered: 'Watch his knuckles, they'll go white.' A consultant psychiatrist for older peoples' services had just been challenged about a local policy. Building up to a crescendo of rage the consultant dominated proceedings for the next five minutes; fists clinched, his knuckles went white. He had two consultant colleagues, one of whom it was rumoured had a car purchased with drug company monetary bonuses. All three of them liked electroshocking old people.

Another research-minded colleague working in adult services (before the days when service commissioners noticed that 'older people' might also be adults) was also an advocate of electroshock. He had noticed that his patients didn't seem much helped by electrocution and suggested a joint research project. Simple stuff: an A-B-A design wherein people were to be asked their current perceptions of mood, randomly allocated electroshock or nothing but chats with the consultant and then asked about their mood again six months later.

The research proposal twice failed to get past the local ethics committee. In common with many other similar research schemes, our study was considered unethical in 'denying' electroshock to the control group of patients inscribed as depressed.

I was once advised that I should write to some eminent UK clinical psychologists with details of an article to be written about what I knew of the great and good of UK clinical psychology. I had taught on most UK doctoral courses and entered the confidence of many senior figures in the profession. I didn't write the article (there's still time), but it was clear that revelations of infidelity, venality and greed might be embarrassing. None of the proposed clinical psychologists had shown me anger. The key feature – for me – of previous clashes with psychiatrists has been anger. Banishment from a ward (see Opposition and Oprah Winfrey) repeating a punishment already witnessed at St John's Hospital, Lincoln during my training (see Bystanders and Bud Powell) was one establishment tactic.

I was less prepared for the consultant psychiatrist who threw a copy of *Toxic Psychiatry* at me when I suggested she read it. I had been taken aback to discover a Lincolnshire psychiatrist who, too drunk to drive, would just leave his car wherever it happened to roll to a halt (including, memorably, at a set of traffic lights in the town adjacent to the psychiatric institution where we both worked) and just as surprised when a psychiatrist colleague revealed he had been on Prozac for years; he didn't much favour electroshock but liked prescribing anti-depressants.

Psychiatrists are overwhelmed with caseloads consisting of people they can't possibly help; partly because there is nothing wrong with them other than their lives and in part because the kind of commitment and resources necessary to change suffering are beyond the power of a single psychiatrist. Many are immersed in a system dependent on Big Pharma and its associated sponsored research articles and many are ordinary folk who find themselves bound up in a system where the pressures of 'clinical responsibility' can only be assuaged by money in the form of research funding or goods. Many are frustrated in their roles and possibly suppressing a good deal of anger just to get through the day. And money, like power corrupts. As Frank Zappa said: '... money ... and that's all we really care about (*it's the thing that sort of sets us apart from the Communists*).'[2]

The global pharmaceuticals market is worth US$400 billion a year, a figure expected to rise to US$500 billion within three years. The ten largest drug companies control over one-third of this market, several with sales of more than US$10 billion a year and profit margins of about 30 per cent. Six are based in the USA and four in Europe.[3]

The National Institute of Health (NIH) is the US government's centre for medical research on humans. Its studies can affect the commercial viability of new drugs and the stock prices of biomedical companies. A decision was made in 1995 by the NIH director to lift restrictions on NIH employees paid for outside consulting. NIH employees were authorized to accept company stock as compensation for consulting. It was later suggested that the NIH could adopt restrictions in place at the FDA, where employees are prohibited from owning stock in companies that may be affected by the agency's decisions.

In 2011, the chairman of the Appropriations Subcommittee on Labour, Health and Human Services and Education asked if ongoing consulting contracts for all NIH employees could be suspended. He noted that various policies and decisions exempted over 90 per cent of the NIH's highest-paid employees from having to publicly disclose payments from drug companies or

235

other outside employers. Officials at the NIH stopped accepting consulting fees and stock options from drug companies later that year.[4]

It is not illegal to pay doctors for promotional work. ProPublica, an independent, non-profit newsroom producing 'investigative journalism in the public interest ...' compiled a list of 384 physicians (out of 17,700 individuals receiving payments) and healthcare providers who earned more than US$100,000 each from one or more of the seven companies disclosing payments in 2009 and early 2010. Nearly all were physicians, 43 of whom were paid more than US$200,000, including two who were paid US$300,000.

More psychiatrists are listed in the database than any other kind of specialist. Of the 384 physicians in the US$100,000 group, 116 are psychiatrists. A psychiatrist based in Chicago, Illinois, received US$203,936 from Eli Lilly, AstraZeneca, Johnson & Johnson and Pfizer, mostly for professional education programmes. A Michigan psychiatrist specializing in child and adolescent psychiatry and forensic psychiatry received over US$200,000, as did an Ohio psychiatrist specializing in addiction psychiatry, forensic psychiatry, geriatric psychiatry, pain medicine and psychosomatic medicine.

Psychiatrists from most American states, including Texas, New York and Utah, feature on the list.[5] There is a fairly lukewarm debate about whether paying doctors to market drugs or publish on electroshock can influence what they prescribe. Gifts and payments, however, are likely to be seen to affect physician's attitudes in much the same way as politicians are regularly accused of financial conflicts of interest or corrupt practices.

As long ago as 1993, it was calculated US psychiatrists could earn an additional $150,000 per annum by giving electroshock to five patients three times a week, '...a target that could easily be achieved in a few hours.'[6]

In the UK, 'payment' can be via conference fees and Pharma-funded meals featuring promotional films, computer equipment and other goods. Any visit to a GP surgery will reveal the overwhelming presence of drug company literature and other promotional material (like the ubiquitous 'drug company pens'). Patients seeking amelioration of distress may not be in the best position to make links between their concerns and the particular drug they are prescribed, even if they notice that the name of the drug manufacturer is emblazoned on the doctor's pen.

Were a patient to make the link, the illness discourse governing the consultation makes it unlikely that anything other than a form of 'illness' will be inscribed and a drug 'treatment' prescribed. As noted previously, once an inscription is made, a referral to a psychiatrist and a recommendation for electroshock may follow.

Opportunities for pharmaceutical companies to offer financial and other incentives are not limited to psy professionals. Under the headline 'NHS fails to declare drug firm cash'. *The Times* summarised an article in the

British Medical Journal: 'Pharmaceutical giants have bought tickets to sports matches and pop concerts for NHS officials as well as sponsoring training events and meetings ... only £1,283,767 of £5,027,818 paid from 2015-2017 was declared on public registers.'

Specifically, local clinical commissioning groups (CCGs) were targeted. CCGs are charged by government with the task of purchasing local health services. Commissioning is governed by NHS England whose guidance was revised after an investigation in 2015 found that £2.4 billion had been paid by CCGs 'to companies, hospitals and surgeries in which their members had financial or professional stakes.' Donations from Pharmaceutical companies between 2015 and 2017 ranged from a £75 ticket to an England cricket match to a subsidy of £24,000 from Bayer, Boehringer Ingelheim and Pfizer for a project in the London Borough of Southwark.[7]

Max Fink was born in Vienna in 1923. He was board certified in neurology in 1952 and psychiatry in 1954 and in 1962 was appointed research professor of psychiatry at Washington University. A decade later, he was appointed professor of psychiatry and neurology at SUNY at Stony Brook. Early research included federal government-funded research into the changes in brain waves (electroencephalogram) induced by electroshock, antidepressant and antipsychotic drugs, opiates and narcotic antagonists, cannabis and metabolites.

Fink has specialized in electroshock research for half a century, during which time his ideas have changed from an early suggestion that the biochemical basis of electroshock is similar to that of craniocerebral trauma through to statements that organic mental syndrome is seen in all patients following shock but is usually transient and finally to the position that treatment-induced memory loss is a hysterical symptom.

In 1985, Fink founded the journal *Convulsive Therapy* (now called the *Journal of ECT*). He was a member of the American Psychiatric Association's task forces on ECT 1975-1978 and 1987-1990.

Fink's awards include the Electroshock Research Association Award (1956), the Laszlo Meduna Prize of the Hungarian National Institute for Nervous and Mental Disease (1986), and Lifetime Achievement Awards of the *Psychiatric Times* (1995) and of the Society of Biological Psychiatry (1996). Publications include *Electroshock: restoring the mind* (1999, Oxford University Press) and, with Jan-Otto Ottosson, *Ethics in electroconvulsive therapy* (2004, Brunner Routledge). In 2007, he funded a book on the history of electroshock by Edward Shorter and David Healy.[8]

Douglas Cameron of the World Association of Electroshock Survivors suggests that the APA Task Force report on electroshock from 1990 might '... more appropriately be deemed The Manufacturers' Task Force Report.' Max Fink was a member of the task force and admitted to receiving royalties from videos marketed by the electroshock device manufacturer Somatics.

Richard Adams, a psychiatrist and the most frequently referenced author in the report owns Somatics while Richard Weiner and Harold Sackheim, both members of the task force, appeared in a video made in 1987 for MECTA (another device manufacturer) *Health Information Network*.[9]

For recipients and for those asking for incarceration or electroshocking of their dependents, vested interest can be financial, for example, when seeking power of attorney over an elderly relative's possessions. The belief that electroshock has been helpful motivates others to undergo it again or opt for 'maintenance ECT' (see Opposition and Oprah Winfrey).

That belief may be held in the face of evidence for the equal effectiveness of sham electroshock (see Marketing and Movies). Being persuaded that the procedure will be a 'life-saver' features in the acceptance of electroshock by suicidal people or the relatives of a suicidal person. A less benign view might be that some people feel they deserve or enjoy punishment while others – particularly parents – are just fed up with their wayward and recalcitrant children (see Youngsters).

Incarceration and electroshock serve the vested interests of shock device manufacturers, psychiatrists, researchers, patients who prefer being inscribed to acknowledging choice for their conduct and parents who want a (marginally) easier life or at least a way of life they imagined before they had children.

Vaslav Nijinsky

In the pre-World War I years, Vaslav Nijinsky lived openly as Diaghilev's lover; they shared hotel suites.

In 1917, after breaking with Diaghilev over his

marriage to Romola (following a two week courtship), Nijinsky moved to St Moritz. He never danced again. Around January 1919, he started retreating to his studio all night long, producing drawing after drawing, at furious speed. The drawings were mostly of eyes. When Romola asked him what they represented, he replied that they were soldiers' faces. 'It is the war,' he said.

One day he went down to St Moritz with a large gold cross over his necktie and stopped people on the street, telling them to go to church. He was occasionally violent; he drove his sleigh into oncoming traffic and threw Romola (holding his daughter Kyra) down a flight of stairs.

In 1919, he was inscribed as schizophrenic by Bleuler and in 1938 was given insulin shocks by Sakel in Bellevue, a nerve clinic run by the Binswanger family.

The pianist Vladimir Horowitz provides a contrast. Horowitz withdrew from many public performances for a decade. After his death, his obituary noted that he had had a successful course of electroshock before his final return to the stage and successful performances at the White House and in Russia and Japan.

A similar argument for the lack of long term negative impact of electroshock could be made on behalf of Lou Reed (see Law and Lou Reed). Despite the electroshock at Creedmore, he went on to become an icon of the bisexual and music communities.

Women

Men do not have a right to assault women or treat them without respect. Men's rights over women have supposedly been reduced since the days of Ancient Greece when women were not regarded as citizens or the millennia old customs of foot-binding in China and genital mutilation all over the world. The practice of *sati* (ritual suicide), where a Hindu widow joins her dead husband on a funeral pyre, was finally outlawed throughout India in 1861. Even so, there were 30 cases of *sati* or attempted *sati* over a 44-year period between 1943 and 1987.[1]

In Australia, during the height of the eugenics movement in the 1920s and 1930s, vast numbers of children of the First Peoples were removed from their families and sent into 'care'. By 1921, 81 per cent of the recorded children removed were girls and girls continued to be disproportionately represented by 1939.[2]

Female rape has been a form of terror used by competing armies; in effect, used as a weapon of war. For the victors, rape – often followed by murder – is a 'spoil' of victory. Genghis Khan is said to have fathered at least 4,000 children by raping the women of conquered tribes. The practice continues in the genocidal wars in the Democratic Republic of the Congo and Rwanda.

In the UK, attitudes to female rape still lean towards a victim-blaming stance. Nearly 15 per cent of respondents to a UK survey thought a woman would be partly responsible for being raped if she was known to have many sexual partners, and 8 per cent saw her as totally responsible. One in three people believes that women who behave flirtatiously are at least partially responsible if they are raped. A similar number think that women are partially or wholly responsible for being raped if they are drunk, and more than a quarter believe women are responsible if they wear 'sexy' or revealing clothing. [3]

The position of women in relation to physical treatments in psy should thus be contextualised within the wider position of women and those who identify as women in society.

The consistent over-representation of women receiving electroshock has frequently been 'explained' in terms of larger numbers of women being inscribed depressed. In many countries, however, those labelled with schizophrenia make up the largest proportion of recipients.[4] A second explanatory discourse emphasizes the relative longer lives of women; as electroshock is more frequently given to older people, there are more women in the target group.

Other tentative hypotheses might include a more general antagonism to women from the male-dominated psy complex or, more radically, the possibility that 'depression' is identified in a group who are actually exhausted by their multiple societal roles and who have less support for their travails. So-called symptoms of depression include early-waking, difficulty in sleeping and feelings about not being good enough and defeated. A common justification for prescribing anti-depressants to people is that they will help the person sleep. This is not always the case but the message is clear: 'You need some rest.'

'Exhaustion' is a normal state for people tasked with caring for and perpetually monitoring children. Mothers may have children by age 12 in some parts of India and in Africa girls may, aged seven, be looking after the remnants of a family devastated by AIDS. In addition to childcare, parents in the industrial areas of the globe may be wage-earning or employed in other ways to maintain a family, potentially looking after ageing family members, carrying out or supervising house-hold duties such as cooking, cleaning or laundering and other activities regarded as essential for survival and maintaining cultural capital.

Such roles are taken by male and female parents in one-parent or multiple care-giver families. 'Traditional' roles of male and female parents are – to an extent – mythic though the expected (*pace* Foucault) performance of men and women can be detected in mass media portrayals of 'exceptional' women who have high profile careers either alongside the parental role or having 'sacrificed' family life.

Women are in the majority of volunteer and unpaid roles; running mother-and-toddler groups, collectivist child nurseries, after school clubs, acting as unpaid secretaries for youth sports organizations, scheduling childcare for school events, participating in 'college-friends' meetings, organizing hospital appointments, meals-on-wheels and other care as low paid care-agency workers, working in charity shops or for furniture and other goods exchange schemes, and so on. Surveys consistently show that in male-female couples the woman will have responsibility for budgeting whether or not she is the principle wage-earner. Virtually any identity or combination of identities – single, lesbian, oppressed, domestic goddess/slave, dutiful/resentful daughter, independent, academic, divorced, monogamous /polygamous, careerist, underpaid or paid less than men doing similar work and so on is held up to scrutiny; and being scrutinized is also exhausting.

Women in the industrialized world lie under the glare of the panopticon and thus the gaze of psy more than men (see Governmentality and Gene Tierney). Further, as noted in Consent and Clementine Churchill and Zealotry and Zelda Fitzgerald, women who find themselves in wholly supportive roles or competitive rather than collaborative relationships with men tend to get the worst deal when it comes to psy intervention.

Karlene Faith sees psychiatry, quite simply, as a tool in the gender politics of the era. After women's suffrage in the United States was guaranteed by the ratification of the Nineteenth Amendment, they ceased to be second-class citizens and began to assert their independence. The male establishment used mental institutions in an effort to disempower them in common with other unmanageable women (see Zealotry and Zelda Fitzgerald).[5] The politics of gender are starkly illustrated in US surveys suggesting that 12 per cent of male and only 3 per cent of female psychologists admit to sex with patients and 13 per cent admit to sex with three or more. In a national survey of American psychiatrists, similar results were found though of 5,574 questionnaires, only 1,423 were returned, of which only 1,316 answered the sexual contact question. The survey was confidential, which begs the question why the other 107 didn't respond.[6]

Bonnie Burstow estimates that 90 per cent of shock doctors are men and in every country where electroshock is used, women are shocked two to three times as often as men, and women over 60 are singularly targeted, accounting for half the statistics. This is despite research demonstrating that older women sustain the most damage.[7] She summarizes electroshock as state sponsored violence against women.[8]

In Victoria, Australia between 2001 and 2008, 18,000 electroshock treatments were reported, 12,000 in the public health system. Of these 18,000, 6,197 shock treatments were compulsory, and nearly three times as many women had shock treatment compared with men.[9]

In California between 1989 and 1994 (1993 figures were unavailable), over 12,000 people received electroshock; about half were over 65 years old, 21 (1.7%) were under 18, and 68 per cent were female.[10] Of the 15,240 shock administrations between September 1993 and April 1995 in Texas hospitals, 70.3 per cent were women.[11]

In England in 2011/2012, around 1,000 people were given electroshock without consent. Over 85 per cent of these were women.[12] In Scotland, according to the Scottish ECT Accreditation Network, 418 patients received electroshock in 2010. The commonest 'indication for treatment' was the failure of prescribed antidepressants (63%). SEAN reported that 75 per cent of patients 'showed an improvement' after a course of electroshock (on average eight treatments). Two thirds of recipients were women.[13]

A review of electroshock use in a group of English NHS trusts between 2011 and 2015 found that two-thirds of recipients were women; 56 per cent of recipients were people aged over 60. The annual dataset released by the Royal College of Psychiatrists shows that for 2016–17, two thirds of patients receiving acute courses of electroshock were female; 74 per cent receiving maintenance electroshock (a procedure supposed to reduce the chances of relapse – see Opposition and Oprah Winfrey) were women; the mean age of patients was 61 for acute shock, and 66 for maintenance.

John Read, professor of clinical psychology at the University of East London, and author of the review said: 'ECT does not tackle the social issues behind why more women than men appear to have depression', and '[ECT] is part of over-medicalising of human distress.'[14]

As noted above, however, (see also Killing with Kindness and Kitty Dukakis), the social issues (and roles) for oppressed and exhausted women are actually transparent. A reduction in the numbers of women inscribed as depressed would require men to relinquish and share some of their power. Further, the possibility that older women in the psy system are the victims of straightforward misogyny should not be ignored (see Sadism and Spike Milligan).

For the human brain, signs of damage are frequently functional. Few psychiatrists or psychiatric nurses will have seen a patient post-electroshock without disturbances in vision, balance or co-ordination. The majority of electroshock nurses, sometimes trained in general as well as psychiatric nursing, are women but, nonetheless, employed in secondary roles without the power to protest on behalf of their 'sisters.' Many will have witnessed in shock survivors post-treatment memory loss of over six months.

The loss of memory is of less concern to clinicians when recipients are women over sixty; symptoms may be interpreted as features of normal ageing. Thus age as well as the supposed psychiatric disorder can be used to distract relatives, carers and patients from iatrogenic sequelae.

Recent years have seen an increase in women prepared to speak out about predatory and assaultive men including other family members and figures in the music, film, sports and fashion industries. Speaking out requires support and a society prepared to listen.[15] An argument can be made for an equally sustained collective vocalization on behalf of women likely to be electroshocked because they are inscribed as depressed rather than oppressed.

For keepers of pauper lunatic houses,

superintendents of insane asylums, alienists and psychiatrists, women's bodies have never been their own. Hundreds of thousands of women have been experimented upon by electroshock doctors and lobotomists. Millions continue to be guinea pigs for pharmaceutical companies, their bodies the sites for internal biochemical warfare.

France Rozier's *Of Secret Habits, or the Ills produced by Onanism in Women* was first published in 1830. For some historians of psychiatry, this willingness on the part of men to pronounce on and interfere with the habits and bodies of perfectly formed females reached its nadir with the case of Isaac Baker-Brown who, '... in the mid 1860s took it into his head that he had discovered the surgical answer to epilepsy, mania and other forms of insanity.'[16]

At the London Surgical Home in Notting Hill, London which he founded, Baker-Brown claimed high rates of success for cures of 'mental disease' via clitoridectomy. Further, Baker-Brown carried out the procedure without the women's consent, a fact finally brought to light in December 1866 when he removed a woman's clitoris during an operation for an anal fissure on the grounds it would prevent her masturbating.

The 1860s were the high point of associating masturbation with insanity though the notion persists to this day.[17] For contemporary psychiatrists, onanism and masturbation are positioned as healthy – a release of pent-up frustration, a way of maintaining arousal in relationships (especially when mutual) and as a means to 'curing' erectile incompetence. This inverts theories prominent in the nineteenth century while illustrating one way in which 'scientific discovery' tends more to a circular than a linear trajectory.

Both Rush in the USA and Esquirol in France regarded masturbation as pathogenic. Both invoked masturbation as a symptom of mania that might, among other possibilities, lead to vertigo, epilepsy and death. Since the 1960s, therapists have suggested this supposed pathogen as a treatment. This is perhaps the equivalent of offering in a few years' time cigarette-smoking as a cure to cancer sufferers or the recent proposal that cannabinol oil might relieve the symptoms of schizophrenia; a reversal of popular theorising that smoking cannabis *leads to* psychosis.[18]

For David Cooper, 'Orgasm is a contagious, good madness.'[19] Cooper adds that orgasm is a political act; the five or so seconds before orgasm are the only time that we are lifted beyond the demands of capitalism. Coming is the only imperative.

Baker-Brown was investigated by the Lunacy Commission (on the grounds that his premises were not licensed to receive those of unsound mind) and in April 1867 was stripped of his fellowship of the Obstetrical Society. Clitoridectomy did not disappear and was still carried out to prevent masturbation and nymphomania in the 1890s. In 1892, Morris, a New York physician published a paper advocating female circumcision in Western women as 80 per cent of 'Aryan American' women suffered from clitoral 'adhesions'. Neuroses, nymphomania, epilepsy and masturbation could be cured through a separation of the adhesion.[20]

Contemporary readers may be appalled by these histories, but actions and reactions are context specific. Baker-Brown and Morris were practicing some sixty years before women in England and America gained the vote, independence in married middle class women was seen as certifiable and husbands had rights close to property rights over their spouses.

Perhaps in sixty years' time, psy historians will be equally taken aback by the wholesale electrocution of millions since 1938.

X-rays

Radiation is linked to psy in two primary ways; as a treatment and as a means of investigating the iatrogenic effects of treatment (bone breakages).

So-called treatments in psychiatry are all a form of magic. The first sleight of hand is to claim that suffering or problematic conduct is an illness. After that, debates about how to 'treat' a 'condition' follow naturally. It's like asking a child if she prefers this or that bed-time story without dropping the idea of 'bed-time'. Parents ask (or tell) their kids to go to bed when they've had enough. Shock doctors prescribe electroshock when they've had enough – a sign of their own limitations rather than a sign there's anything wrong with the patient that can't be fixed by just waiting.

At the turn of the nineteenth and twentieth centuries, science was in the ascendant, the industrial revolution had given way to what might be called the industrial era and advances were being proclaimed in numerous areas of human endeavour, from vaccination to printing via increasingly efficient transport systems based on steam engines. H.G. Wells had inspired the populace with *The First Men in the Moon*, and powered flight, telecommunication and the motor car were all on the visible horizon. Any group wishing for prestige and public appeal needed to appeal to the popularity of science.

Electricity was beginning to buzz around and radio-activity was already known. What better way to inspire confidence in up-to-the-minute scientistic endeavour than to use both?

Uranium was discovered by German chemist Martin Klaproth in 1789. A century later in November 1895 Roentgen discovered the x-rays of uranium. By February the following year, they were in medical use in the USA. Two years later Marie Curie (the only woman to have won the Nobel Prize twice) named the properties of her newly discovered radium radioactivity. Within a few years radiation therapy was being hailed as a treatment for cancer.

Radium Therapy for those with psy inscriptions began in the early 20th century. There had been experiments with radium to treat epilepsy (a common reason for incarceration in an asylum) and the theories of Julius Nyirö soon led to experimentation on those labelled schizophrenic (see History and Hemingway). Solutions of free radium salts were available; the salts could be added to baths or directly applied to the body, externally and internally via every orifice.

X-rays are implicated in psycho-surgery. In 1908 Spiegel (a neurologist) and Wycis (a neurosurgeon) were the first to use x-rays in stereotaxic (now stereotactic) surgery. The patient's brain was x-rayed and then air injected into the ventricles to provide spatial coordination for ablation (destruction) of brain cells. Anterior capsulotomy has been used for people inscribed as obsessive-compulsive in the UK and Sweden, and Anterior cingulotomy for 'cases of anxiety, depression and obsessive compulsive disorder.'

First discovered in 1794, Yttrium (commonly used in cases of liver cancer) is still used in Stereotactic Subcaudate Tractotomy for those in Korea inscribed with OCD. For all these interventions limbic leucotomy to produce up to 14 cryogenic lesions in the brain is the next step if previous surgery has failed.[1] Developed in 1973 by Desmond Kelly and surgeon Alan Richardson at Atkinson Morley's Hospital a 50 per cent success rate was originally claimed for the procedure.

In the years immediately following the First World War, Henry Cotton's pursuit of focal infection as the root of insanity necessitated a full dental suite and x-ray equipment (see Torture). Cotton was keen to merge essentially descriptive psychopathology of the nineteenth century with the physical realities of medical science and ensure that his approach was seen to be as modern as possible. To that extent his diagnostic efforts involved bacteriological and serological investigation and the new magic of x-rays: 'Even 'apparently toothless' patients needed careful scrutiny with X-rays, lest they have some remaining impacted or unerupted molar lurking unseen to perpetuate their madness.'[2]

The search for 'disease' has not been limited to Cotton's arcane methods. Luxenburg and colleagues used x-ray computer tomography to isolate brain abnormalities in patients inscribed with OCD.[3] Such searches cannot succeed due to the metaphoric nature of psy conditions, but they are invariably flawed because patients will have been prescribed many different psycho-active drugs that will impact on the brain. Any brain changes are likely to be iatrogenic in origin.[4]

Paradoxically, radiation therapy has not only been proposed as a 'cure' for psy recipients, it has been implicated as a causal agent in distress defined as disease. For example, one study looked at 177 cases treated 10-29 years earlier for ringworm of the scalp by x-ray therapy or by chemotherapy. The irradiated group manifested more inscribable behaviours and more deviant MMPI (*Minnesota Multiphasic Personality Inventory*) scores. They were also judged more maladjusted from their MMPI profiles, and more frequently had a history of treated psychiatric disorders.[5]

Most recently, x-rays have been used as an example of exaggerated fear of those inscribed as obsessive-compulsive. The author's own position on the safety of x-rays is authoritative and dismissive of peoples' fears:

'The X-rays from a single chest X-ray or from dental X-rays are trivial. Yet some patients with OCD treat all radiation as if it is deadly. Consider this: radon, which is a radioactive breakdown product of uranium, is present in every basement to a varying degree, usually in very small amounts. Since patients with OCD cannot reliably estimate risk, I suggest to them that they rely on the judgement of others, particularly experts.'

His patients have a response: 'They retort by telling

me that experts can be found on every side of an issue.'[6]

Succinylcholine-modified electroshock was introduced over fifty years ago as a means of avoiding broken bones so prevalent during electrocution, a procedure that necessitated the use of x-rays post-shock. Nevertheless, unmodified shock continues to be practiced. It has been suggested that unmodified shock is still practiced because it takes less time to administer and is 'more convenient' than modified electroshock.

In its resource book on mental health, human rights, and legislation, the World Health Organization addresses unmodified electroshock in two sentences, stating that its practice should be stopped. The World Psychiatric Association (WPA) position statement on unmodified electroshock has asked national member societies to implement modified shock as the standard, placing the responsibility for this directive on governments, professional organizations, and individual practitioners (see Governmentality and Gene Tierney). The American Psychiatric Association and the Royal College of Psychiatrists offer no comments on unmodified electroshock and assume that electroshock is always modified.

Despite these strictures, unmodified electroshock has been reported from Nigeria, Uganda, the United Kingdom, France, Spain, Russia, Japan, China and Turkey (see Torture). Chanpattana and Kramer reported that 94 per cent of electroshock in Thailand was unmodified.[7] In a French study, only 5 of 75 patients received modified shock series and in Spain, 5 per cent of units never administered a muscle relaxant and 3 per cent did so only occasionally.

As noted previously (see, for example, Death-making and David Reville) electroshock can be destructive to memory, life and limb. The advent of modified electroshock with the use of anaesthesia massively reduced the likelihood of fractures (to the neck, ribs and scapulae) to the recipient. Even so, Kalinowsky, who reported a death rate of up to one in a 1,000 recipients, suggested that it was anaesthesia techniques rather than electrocution that increased the fatalities.[8]

With the exception of those countries in the paragraph above and 'emergency' shock where anaesthesia is unavailable, the need for x-rays post-shock has markedly reduced. The possibilities of radiation as a treatment are likely to continue to be explored in a system where magic and scientism go hand in hand.

Youngsters

For people in their sixties, anyone under thirty is likely to be seen as a 'youngster.' For the purposes of this chapter, the term refers to infants, children and adolescents; still an age range of twenty years with varying definitions and understandings of each grouping.

Abraham was prepared to sacrifice Isaac to Jehovah and parents have offered up their children – literally and metaphorically – to various authorities ever since. Frequently this is justified in terms of what's 'best' for the child; circumcision, sending a child away to boarding school and spanking are all carried out in the 'child's best interests'. The dominance of parents over their offspring is a feature of myth, literature and reality.

Cronos ate all his new-born children until the birth of Zeus, Romulus and Remus were abandoned by their father Amulius to die in the Tiber, and Herod killed all the male children of Jews in his hunt for the baby Jesus. *Hansel and Gretel* and *The Water Babies* were popular stories in Victorian England. Children have always been sold into slavery. In 1885, for example, in order to prove that white slavery was a thriving industry, W. T. Stead of the *Pall Mall Gazette* was arrested for buying a 13-year-old girl in Marylebone, London.[1] The practice continues to hit the UK press headlines with some regularity.

Children still living at home are dependent on their parent(s) for protection. If a parent cannot cope with a child's conduct, there are several options; from literal abandonment to seeking expert help. The *DSM5* lists numerous possible inscriptions available for use by psy professionals should the youngster's behaviour prove sufficiently disturbing to powerful others. Inscribed children have a higher chance of being medicated or given electroshock though the child's lack of power means that no inscription is necessary for psy involvement (see Consent and Clementine Churchill) as 'Poverty, untreatability, chance and the desire to escape punishment, rather than need for medical attention are often the tickets of entry to child psychiatric services.'[2]

Most frequently children enter psy services because a parent wants them to. To an extent, in the UK, psy institutions (frequently called 'units') and social service run children's homes have replaced the places where nineteenth century unwanted children wound up: prisons, workhouses, epileptic colonies, insane asylums and orphanages. Twenty years ago in the USA, hundreds of thousands of children were housed in psychiatric facilities despite the fact that 'three quarters of the children had no psychotic symptoms...'[3]

Szasz's summary of this state of affairs is cogent: 'Child psychiatry *is* child abuse.'[4]

Child and adolescent services are ambiguous concerning their definition of childhood. In the UK NHS, different regions and health administrative structures differ in their definitions of the points at which a child becomes an adolescent and then an adult. For some, the definitions depend on education; a child becomes an adolescent when she enters secondary education, becoming an adult when she leaves the school system. For others there are age demarcations; 'children' remain children until age 13 and are adolescents until, roughly, 20 making adolescents within the definition teenagers.

In other services 'children' effectively become 'adults' if child services cannot cope – many patients have been admitted, aged 10, to psychiatric hospitals since the nineteenth century. US asylums had so many children behind their walls that a new discipline of inpatient child psychiatry began by default. In the middle of the nineteenth century Bellevue Asylum in New York held over 1,000 children under the age of 16.[5,6]

Beyond the confines of structuralised service definitions, for many parents their children remain 'children' all their lives. Parents may still refer to sons as 'boys' or daughters as 'girls' long past the point their offspring have reached adulthood.

For parents whose offspring never leave home or, due to being marked as 'disabled' have been institutionalised, the social context re-languages the child as 'lazy', 'dependent', or, in the case of those with physical disabilities or psy inscription, 'eternally innocent' or 'tragic'. Service definitions of childhood reflect wider societal ambiguities: in the UK, a 10-year-old can be tried for murder, but that same child would have to wait until 16 to legally begin a consensual sexual relationship, 17 to drive, 18 to vote, and so on. In the USA, the age demarcation lines differ between states for driving, owning a gun and buying alcohol. The brain, however, continues to develop throughout adolescence. For neurologists, it is undisputed that the developing brain is vulnerable; any assault on brain tissue – whether it be biochemical, traumatic or through electroshock – is injurious to brain cells and neuronal connections.

In 1947, child neuropsychiatrist Lauretta Bender (to become famous as the progenitor of the Bender-Gestalt test) published a study carried out on 98 children aged between four and 11 years old who had been treated in the previous five years with intensive courses of electroshock. Most were inscribed with 'childhood schizophrenia'. These children received shock daily for a typical course of approximately 20 treatments,[7] an intensive regime first suggested by Bini and known as regressive ECT or annihilation therapy.[8] Beneficial effects of electroshock were reported in the majority but complete remission was rare.

Bender abandoned the use of electroshock in the 1950s. Her published work was discredited after a study showing that the children had either not improved or had been harmed.[9] During the 1960s, Bender supervised the children's unit of Creedmoor Hospital (see: Law and Lou Reed and Bystanders and Bud Powell). It has been described as a 'veritable snake pit'.[10] Her assessment technique consisted of an interview with the child, followed by analysis of the child's responses and conduct in front of a large group

261

of staff and the child, as though the latter could not hear. The technique bears comparison with the earlier work of Gessel (see Governmentality and Gene Tierney), work that made the child the object of study and inscription as if the researchers were irrelevant.

Bender performed a 'diagnostic test' on children, which involved holding the head of a standing child and gently turning it. Supposedly, schizophrenic children would turn in the direction of the pressure and normal children would resist.[11] Her praxis is almost archetypal in its portrayal of the lack of objective science that characterises psy (see Precision and Mervyn Peake).

Research on electroshock with children is bedevilled by methodological, ethical and philosophical questions. As noted elsewhere psy inscription (diagnosis) is both unreliable and invalid. The practice depends on notions of interiority and individuality that are impossible to verify by the methods of science. Nonetheless research is ubiquitous for reasons outlined in Research and Robeson.

Rey and Walter discuss an example of a 15-year-old girl inscribed with schizophrenia who received 200 electroshocks in one year. More dramatically, they cite a 16-year-old girl inscribed with dementia praecox who was given 15 unmodified electroshocks in three days. She developed an organic brain syndrome over a period of three weeks. Five other patients were reported to have ended the shock treatment prematurely due to adverse effects.

These included a depressed teenager who was considered 'manic' after five shocks, two whose treatment was discontinued because of increasing agitation, one who showed marked confusion after two treatments and an 18-year-old inscribed with bipolar disorder who developed neuroleptic malignant syndrome following one session.[12]

Writing in *Convulsive Therapy*, Cohen and colleagues reviewed the medical records of 21 children aged between 13 and 19 who had been given bilateral electroshock from 1984 to 1995. They found a 40 per cent relapse rate after a year. Partial 'clinical improvement' occurred for some 'schizophrenic and schizoaffective episodes'. Adverse effects were transient but 'frequent'. The researchers concluded that 'ECT is a safe and effective treatment for adolescents with severe and intractable mental illness.'[13]

As half of the recipients relapsed and adverse effects were acknowledged as frequent, this seems a conservative reading of the data. The conclusion exactly mimics promotional literature from both the American Psychiatric Association and Britain's Royal College of Psychiatrists. Numerous studies and reviews come to a similar conclusion.[14] Wachtel and colleagues suggest that 'the indications for electroconvulsive therapy in children and adolescents are similar to those in adults, including severe affective, psychotic and catatonic pathology'.

Arguing that it is bad publicity that prevents clinicians and parents considering shock as an option, they urge the 'removal of impediments to ECT access in this population', adding that children diagnosed with autism and neurodevelopmental disabilities should also be candidates.[15]

A further study examines shock treatment of a 14-year-old boy labelled with moderate learning disability and autism. His existing catatonic stupor required him to have nasogastric nutrition and fluid replacement. Antidepressants hadn't helped and zolpidem produced only a temporary improvement in the catatonia. The authors conclude that bilateral electroshock 'produced a significant response after the third treatment, and progressive improvement to the end of the course of 13 sessions'.

In a classic example of reverse logic the authors suggest: 'Successful maintenance on a neuroleptic–lithium combination and previous episodes of catatonic excitement are suggestive of an underlying bipolar disorder.'[16] This is not unlike concluding that, because a plaster cast helped a person walk better, she must have had a broken leg when closer examination would have revealed that her legs were tied together.

In Israel, a study compared the results of electroshock in two groups (adolescents and adults) in a community psychiatric institution. The files of 24 consecutive adolescent patients treated in the years 1991 to 1995 were retrospectively examined, and the findings were compared with those for 33 adult patients who started their shock course on the same day. The authors conclude that shock was equally effective for adolescents and adults (58 per cent in each group achieved remission).[17]

Willoughby reports a case study of one 8-year-old girl inscribed with psychotic depression and concludes:

'Nurses and other healthcare personnel should consider ECT in refractory cases of major depressive disorder, bipolar affective disorder, schizophrenia, and other psychotic disorders.'[18]

Comparing shock use in adolescents with shock use in patients of other ages, adolescents subjected to electroshock account for only 0.43 per cent of the total treatments in India, 0.93 per cent in Australia and 1.5 per cent in the USA.[19,20,21] A study from New South Wales involved a 53-item telephone survey with people who received electroshock before the age of 19 years. Opinions were generally positive; the majority considered electroshock a legitimate treatment, would have it again and recommend it to others. Throughout Australia in the year 2007-2008, there were 203 electroshock episodes with children younger than 14 – including 55 carried out on children aged four and younger. Two of the under-fours were in Victoria.[22]

In July 2002, the Brazilian Federal Council of Medicine, in its Resolution n. 1640, regulated the use of electroshock in Brazil. It prohibited the use of shock in patients below 16 years of age, unless in exceptional circumstances.[23] Partly in response to this resolution, Lima and colleagues conducted an extensive review of electroshock use with young people. They define adolescence as the 'state of being 13 to 18 years of age' and surveyed three medical databases: PMC (United States National Library of Medicine), LILACS (Literatura Latino-Americana e do Caribe em Ciências da Saúde), and SciELO (Scientific Electronic Library Online).

The research is something of an object lesson in the academy's demand for publication; there are 16 authors named in a study that was, in effect, a literature search and review. Inclusion criteria were: (1) manuscripts written in English, Portuguese, Spanish or French; (2) case reports, series of cases, case controls, literature reviews, cross-sectional studies, exploratory field research, and prospective and retrospective cohort studies; (3) studies regarding the use of shock in adolescents, provided they respected at least three of the five PICOS criteria: adolescent, ECT, absent or only drugs, symptoms remission, and study design. Studies assessing other conditions, editorials and letters to the editor were excluded.

From the 212 studies surveyed, the authors reduced their final total to 33, a further six being added from research referenced in the reviewed sample.[24] The authors conclude that electroshock use in adolescents is 'considered a highly efficient option for treating several psychiatric disorders, achieving high remission rates, and presenting few and relatively benign adverse effects'.[25] In their introduction, they suggest that adolescents experience 'self-destruction impulses' (The authors do not reflect on the possibility that agreeing to electroshock is, in itself, self-destructive).

The authors note that the American Academy of Child and Adolescent Psychiatry (AACAP) has established that eligibility for electroshock in adolescents involves meeting three criteria: (1) diagnosis, (2) severity of symptoms, (3) lack of treatment response to appropriate psychopharmacological agents accompanied by other appropriate treatment modalities. Electroshock is recommended for adolescents labelled with persistent major depression, schizoaffective disorder, schizophrenia, or history of manic episodes, with or without psychotic features.[26]

Other researchers have suggested that electroshock can be used with children and adolescents to treat catatonia and neuroleptic malignant syndrome.[27,28] The latter is one adverse effect of neuroleptic medication. Here further brain damage is being recommended as a treatment for iatrogenic harm. Notwithstanding the lack of validity in psy inscription, electroshock is most frequently used with children labelled depressed – a supposed 'mood disorder'. It has also been used with children and adolescents inscribed as 'bi-polar', 'mentally retarded', 'autistic', 'schizophrenic', and 'endogenously depressed'. [29,30,31,32,33,34,35] This last illustrates the unreliability of using even relatively recent research to support contemporary treatments in the field; 'endogenous' depression was removed from the official lexicon over 30 years ago.

Lima and colleagues conclude: 'ECT is the treatment of choice depending on diagnosis, severity of symptoms, and lack of response to psycho-pharmacotherapy. The majority of the studies in the scientific literature show the efficiency of ECT use in adolescents and consider this approach more efficient than psychopharmacotherapy isolated [sic].' And 'an experienced staff and adequate physical conditions can minimize the risk of complications.' Iatrogenic harm is thus reduced to 'complications'.[36]

In contrast, Jones and Baldwin remark: 'ECT has been repackaged in a manner designed to censor public opinion. Empirical research, based on adequate methodological data, does not exist.'[37]

The lack of controlled studies is a common concern amongst electroshock reviewers. A recent review of the procedure with children marked as learning disabled found no controlled studies, the majority of articles consisting of case reports. The authors performed an online literature search for national and international journal articles published before March 2010. They found 72 case reports, a retrospective chart review study and other reviews, but no controlled studies.

Despite the lack of rigour, the review suggests that, 'Most patients (79%) showed a positive outcome following ECT. Complications were seen only in 13 per cent and there were no reports of cognitive decline.' Many patients, however, relapsed following electroshock (32%), the majority being medicated at follow-up (71%).[38] Despite these results and concerns that 'the sample is relatively small and there is a definite skew in the severity of intellectual disability represented, with the majority of case reports discussing patients with mild and moderate disability', the authors conclude: 'Electroconvulsive therapy is a valuable treatment for this patient group and should be considered earlier as opposed to as a last resort.'

The identified obstacles to its use noted by the authors include: 'diagnostic difficulties, ethical and legal issues, a lack of objective measurements and uncertainty about its safety in this population'.[39]

Other authors see few ethical challenges:

'If patients with intellectual disability are likely to suffer more because of ... medications and their inability to report somatic side-effects, it may be that ECT would benefit them by reducing the need for multiple medications.'[40]

This reasoning has led others to conclude: 'In specific patients [children inscribed as learning disabled], ECT may actually be the more conservative treatment option'.[41]

Herman and colleagues showed that rates of electroshock use across US states were highly variable, higher than for most medical and surgical procedures. In some urban areas, access to shock is limited. In 13 US states, the procedure is regulated by law and in Colorado and Texas is forbidden for children under 16. In Missouri, a court order is needed. In Tennessee, a child can be electroshocked only for 'mania or severe depression'.[42]

The poor public image of the procedure and 'safe and effective' rhetoric is further addressed in a web-based article; 'ECT in kids: Safe, effective, robust and... underutilized'.[43] The article reports on a 20-year retrospective study by investigators at the Mayo Clinic in Rochester, Minnesota, presented at the American Psychiatric Association's 2013 Annual Meeting.[44] The Mayo is one of the few centres in the United States using electroshock with children and adolescents. The presenters claimed that the procedure reduced 'symptoms of affective disorders, psychotic disorders, and other disorders' up to one year post-treatment with a single series of shocks. They noted that a poor public image and the controversy over its use have led to its subsequent underutilisation and suggested that the image was based on 'outdated misconceptions'.[45]

At the Mayo Clinic, electroshock is carried out under the supervision of an anaesthesiologist as well as a psychiatrist. For the study, the investigators examined the medical records of all patients from the ages of 12 to 19 years treated with shock at the Mayo Clinic from 1993 to 2012. The study included 46 patients for 29 of whom one-year follow-up data were available.

The authors suggest that the majority were 'suffering from severe, recalcitrant, and frequently comorbid mood, anxiety, and psychotic illnesses - with about an even split between recurrent major depressive disorder and primary psychotic disorder. Other disorders included anorexia nervosa, catatonia, and schizoaffective disorder'.

Most recipients were on at least four psychoactive medications simultaneously; the researchers make no causal link between the effects of these medications and the various 'disorders'. The most common adverse effects of electroshock were nausea (15.2%) and headaches (13%), followed by 'post-emergent agitation' (8.7%) and spontaneous seizure (4.3%). The presenters concluded that 'ECT remains the gold standard for severe illness.'[46]

Two, essentially pro-electroshock, studies have

detailed the medical procedures seen as necessary when considering electroshock. The first looked at referred adults and found that they have a greater number of pathological lesions of the central nervous system as identified by a CT or MRI scan. The author suggests that some of these lesions may affect treatment outcome or seizure duration. Therefore, an MRI or CT scan is indicated in adolescents before shock treatment. This is a costly recommendation unlikely to be carried out even by those practitioners who may have read the study.[47]

The second study examined the effectiveness and safety of electroshock in 'pharmacotherapy-refractory depression' in 11 hospitalised adolescents. A potentially serious complication of tardive seizure occurred in one recipient. Prolonged seizures were noted in seven of the 11 patients. Pending further research, the authors recommended that electroshock should only be administered to youth in hospital settings, that all regularly administered psychotropic medications (including antidepressants) be discontinued before shock, and that physicians be aware that 12 treatments are 'usually sufficient'.[48]

It is unknown how many practitioners follow these recommendations. The recommendations, however, remain part of rhetoric consistent with the notion that professionals should be trusted – and may be held to account if not following guidelines claimed to enhance 'safety.' Thomas Szasz has also suggested that the siting of electroshock facilities in general hospitals maintains the illusion that psychiatry is a genuine branch of physical medicine.[49]

For children and adolescents, debate about the use of electroshock is mostly confined to activists, frequently online, and within the pages of psychiatric journals. Research criteria invariably involve the subjects under scrutiny. Criteria for researchers rarely go beyond a brief allusion to their academic qualifications. Research on electroshock, a treatment designed to destroy brain cells, neuronal connections and memory, should, perhaps, include criteria for those very researchers.

Do we know, for example, if the researchers are parents? If they are, do we know if they like children? The scientistic ethos in the psy complex presumes that researchers are neutral observers. It is clear, however, that some people do not like children. Any parent is likely to go through periods of wanting offspring to leave home as soon as possible. Adults who are not parents may regard their lack of offspring as a choice, based on not particularly liking or valuing children. For children and teenagers, there is no guarantee of sympathy from adults and adult researchers. One criterion for shock practitioners might then be to answer, as honestly as possible: 'Why do you think you want to electrocute young people?'

The vested interest would be in profiting through the satisfaction of harming people rather than material gain (the interest declared as a 'conflict of interest' in journal articles). Science demands the most parsimonious theories to explain results. Uncomfortable though it certainly is to contemplate the possibility that psy professionals and parents set out to harm children, this is one hypothesis that might bear further scrutiny.

Children, as minors, are not protected by the law. As Szasz has remarked, when parents are distressed by or don't like their children's behaviour the children are sent to psy professionals – a possibility that becomes increasingly likely as the language of psy becomes ubiquitous. Under the guise of care, parents – frequently supported by teachers and educational psychologists – can ask for a psychiatric intervention having already inscribed a child as ADHD or depressed rather than excitable or moody. The labelling avoids the guilt of implicitly admitting to not being able to cope or, on occasions, just wanting the child to become someone else's responsibility. Szasz adds that many parents do this to avoid scrutiny of their own tempestuous relationship.[50] Of course, many refer out of desperation.

Elsewhere, Robbie Piper, a primary school teacher, has described the guilt he experiences when recommending young children for psy assessment simply because an inscription and subsequent medication will allow him time to focus on more engaged pupils.[51]

Mental health legislation in Western Australia banning the use of electroshock on those under 14 passed through state parliament in October 2014. The law imposes a $15,000 fine on a member of psy electrocuting a child under 14. A child aged between 14 and 18 who is a voluntary patient cannot have the treatment without informed consent and approval by the Mental Health Tribunal.[52]

For many psy professionals, use of electroshock with children is condoned only in extremis and where it might be described as 'life saving'. Some psychiatrists recommend electroshock as the preferred choice of intervention, an argument made on its behalf for older people and in pregnant women. Aziz and colleagues suggest that electroshock should be seen as 'the more conservative option' for people marked as autistic.[53]

Lack of power places minors at risk of a breach of their right to treatment and their right to refuse treatment.[54] They are at greater risk from adult exploitation in clinical and research settings. In either, the imbalance of power might suggest that minors are *de facto* exploited. Baldwin notes that: 'Paradoxically so-called outpatient treatment may be the *most coercive of all interventions*'[55] (emphasis in the original). He gives 'Assertive Community Treatment' and early intervention psychosis programmes in the USA, Australia and the UK as examples of psy interventions that override the fundamental right not to be treated.

The *World Medical Association* 'Declaration of Helsinki' in 1964 included specific direction about consent. For minors consent reverts to the parent(s) or legal guardian(s) *in loco parentis*. For institutionalised minors, the state assumes legal custody *in parens patriae*. For parents acting in the child's best interests, this requires agencies to provide sufficient information for the parent(s) to make a judgement about pursuing treatment. Agencies and psy professionals have been slow to embrace this agenda. For example, a report in 2001 confirmed that parents of children inscribed with ADHD and prescribed methylphenidate (Ritalin) were not informed that the drug is a member of the amphetamine family. Instead, echoing promotional material on electroshock, they were told the drug was 'safe and effective'.

Curiously, parents were informed that Ritalin and similar drugs are 'non-addictive', despite the known addictive qualities of amphetamine.[56] There is an argument here for regarding maintenance electroshock as *addictive* – for recipients and shock practitioners.

Readers may have noted the conflictual conclusions of electroshock researchers. Research repeatedly shows that youngsters are harmed or, in some cases, die as a result of electroshock. Those same thorough reports end by suggesting that electroshock is the preferred intervention for a growing number of inscribed children and adolescents. Although fewer youngsters appear to be receiving electroshock, this expansion of the recommended recipients through broadening the number of inscriptions maintains the overall numbers.

Loretta Bender used electroshock for children inscribed as schizophrenic. For many years, youngsters marked as depressed were the preferred recipients. As 'childhood schizophrenia' faded from the lexicon to be replaced by autism and sad youngsters were increasingly prescribed drugs so a new market had to be found. As noted above, that market now includes just about every unmanageable kid you can think of.

I have described elsewhere how the criteria for a

diagnosis of autism has expanded to involve a 'spectrum' wherein almost any child can lie on the spectrum as it incorporates many behaviours, however undesirable, that are common amongst children.[57] If shock is seen as a first treatment for those marked as autistic, then the following informed consent form may be the way forward for concerned parents and carers:

'Your child has received a psychiatric diagnosis. This label has no validity but may be based on a foreign language so it sounds impressive. Your consultant may or may not like children and has a history of electrocuting them. The electric shocks will destroy brain cells and will have little effect in the long term on the behaviour of your child, who will continue to be medicated with a variety of harmful drugs. There is a chance your child will die from the electric shock or anaesthesia.'

Magic has long been a component of psy theorising and praxis. This magic is contextual and shifts within a wider zeitgeist. Thus counselling, mindfulness, psychopharmacology and other psy interventions rely on mysterious processes and biochemical changes both invisible and unknown involving many competing hypotheses to patients *and* professionals. Appeals to broad constructs such as 'connectedness', 'community', or 'mind' continue alongside more specific notions of 'brain-biochemical imbalance' or 'genetic predisposition'. All such constructs are, by necessity, metaphorical. The language of psy borrows from and lends to a wider discourse of individuality and interiority where 'selves' are constructed and behaviour described in psy terminology by the public as much as by psy experts.

The magic inherent in this discourse involves, in the case of electroshock, a further appeal to the culturally valued tropes of 'science' and 'research'. It is this cultural value, rather than any proven benefit to patients, that will maintain the use of electroshock with children. As experts and the public are less beguiled by the mysteries of electricity, the praxis will, like insulin-coma therapy before it, become an historical footnote in the annuls of psy, of value to publishers and historians who will, perhaps, shock us metaphorically rather than literally.

Almost a century ago, in 1925, Henry Cotton (see Women and X-rays) recommended the screening of all schoolchildren in case they were harbouring an infection that would later lead to psychosis. He regarded 'abnormal childhood sexuality' as evidence of chronic sepsis and toxaemia and performed colectomies as a way to reduce masturbation. Not quite on a par with the likely result of contemporary calls for the screening of US and UK children for signs of mental disorder but equally self-serving and, of course, couched in terms of helping youngsters.[58]

Zealotry
and Zelda Fitzgerald

The first Zealots were members of a Judean Jewish sect who fought to the death against the Romans and who killed or persecuted Jewish collaborators.

The word implies an uncompromising pursuit of religious, political, or other ideals and is a synonym for fanaticism. Kitty Dukakis has been described as an 'evangelist' for electroshock (see Killing with Kindness and Kitty Dukakis). 'Fanatics' are no longer simply fans – of pop icons or artistic figures. The word tends to be associated with terrorism. Terror for many is part of daily experience for people involved in the practice of electroshock. The terrorist can be the psychiatrist threatening to forcibly detain someone unless they agree to be shocked or kindly nurses persuading the patient that 'the treatment is for the best.'

The terrorised are the patients who instinctively (and accurately) know that electric shocks are unlikely to be good for the brain; as noted in Torture, an association between terror and torture is acknowledged in countries like Turkey where electroshock is, indeed, used as a form of torture on young people.

The zealous pursuit of cure in particularly dramatic ways against both the evidence and what common sense might suggest has been a feature of psychiatry since the nineteenth century when high-minded theorizing suggested that electric shocks applied directly to the testicles of runaway slaves would cure them of 'drapetomania' – the desire to run away from benevolent slave-owners.

Protest requires an equal expenditure of energy. For at least ten years, the blog *ECT Statistics* has been regularly updated by one person giving readers information on everything from the most recent theories on electroshock to its practice in Nepal and Peru.[1]

Zealotry was a feature of the career of Walter Freeman, a pioneer of lobotomy. During the Second World War, lobotomy became a preferred treatment for those labelled as obsessive or psychotic. Valenstein, however, has shown that early claims for the cure of patients undergoing the surgery were exaggerated; its earliest user, Egas Moniz, was unable to demonstrate that any of his patients were enabled to live outside the hospital, and death or apathy were common outcomes. Despite this, Lisbon boasts a large statue to Moniz, Portugal's only Nobel Prize winner.

Freeman and Watts had been responsible for a new surgical procedure in 1937, the severing of nerve connections between the frontal lobes and the rest of the cortex. This was the standard lobotomy until Freeman pioneered the trans-orbital lobotomy in 1945. The modified procedure involved inserting an ice pick through the eye socket in order to sever nerve connections. Between 1936 and 1951, over 18,000 lobotomies were performed in the USA.

In December 1940, Golla, at Bristol's Burden

Neurological Unit, performed the UK's first lobotomy. Less than 15 years later, over 12,000 similar operations had been carried out in England and Wales.[2]

Valenstein has extensively researched Freeman's career. His method, to electroshock a patient into unconsciousness before performing the operation, was eventually superseded by the use of anaesthesia. His enthusiasm and dedication were remarkable. In 1951, Freeman visited hospitals in seventeen states and several Canadian provincial hospitals in addition to demonstrating the technique in Puerto Rico and Curaçao.

During that summer he drove 11,000 miles, 'in a station wagon loaded ...with an electroconvulsive box, a Dictaphone, and a file cabinet filled with patient records, photographs, and correspondence; his surgical instruments were in his pocket.' Between the end of June and early August, he performed 111 operations including 25 in one day in Cherokee, Iowa.[3]

To his credit and unlike numerous other members of psy, Freeman spent many years post-retirement on extraordinarily exhausting peregrinations (he was suffering from rectal cancer) following up ex-patients.[4]

The same zealous approach sometimes applies more reflexively as in the case of the medical superintendent and his colleagues at Shropshire's Shelton Hospital in the late 1950s who gave each other shocks (see Justification and Janet Frame). There is also the – possibly – apocryphal tale of a local farmer who bypassed the need for psychiatric authority by giving himself rather haphazard electric shocks via the battery of his tractor.

The stories of Moniz, Freeman, Sakel and Cerletti demonstrate there is room, indeed approbation, for zealotry in inventing novel medical technique. Without passion and commitment and the support of powerful allies, new techniques would never emerge. In the case of lobotomy, enthusiasm waned; but only after thousands of people had been harmed and killed. A much modified version obtains; now involving ablation of brain matter via electrodes.

In a system where certain medical procedures like electroshock are neither publicly discussed nor officially recorded, zealotry can thrive. Electroshock appears to be making a recovery.

Alongside this attachment to electrocution, there has often been a rather shame-faced, almost secretive, attitude to electroshock amongst professionals. For example, despite the shock suite being originally in the entrance corridor of Oxford's Warneford Hospital, for many years it was disguised to visitors by an illuminated sign reading 'Dentist' when in use.

In the late 1990s, a clinical psychologist, on first moving to St George's Hospital in Stafford, found her office located alongside the discrete electroshock suite. She was regularly interrupted by the dimming of her office lights due to fluctuations in electricity when the suite was in use.

Even the use of the term 'suite' has subtle – possibly deliberate – associations. The best rooms in hotels are suites, even (to stretch the point) onomatopoetically – sweet. In the clinic, the term refers to the original arrangement of frequently three rooms: a preparation room, the electroshock room and the 'recovery' room.

As noted in Evidence and Electrocution, secrecy around electroshock extends to record-keeping. In a state system over-burdened with data collection on everything from the number of hip operations carried out annually to the number of toilet rolls ordered, it has become increasingly difficult finding information on the use of electroshock in the UK's NHS of the twenty-first century.

The available figures do suggest, however, that pockets of zealous use of shock exist; in several cases the outcome has been that these facilities are used for referrals from other counties. At an international level, the banning of electroshock in Slovenia has led to Slovenian authorities sending patients to Croatia for electroshock (see Law and Lou Reed). Effectively banned in Italy, Austria, Germany and Switzerland for some years, electroshock is now returning throughout these countries.

Peter Lehmann, a publisher and founder of the European Network of Users and Survivors of Psychiatry, claims that one person, Uwe Peters, recently appointed to the ethical council of the German Society for Psychiatry, Psychotherapy and Neurology, is responsible for the resurgence of electroshock in Germany.[5]

Edward Shorter objects to regulations concerning the use of electroshock with young people that mean children must be moved across state boundaries to be shocked. He claims electroshock is the 'penicillin of psychiatry' and states: 'The legislative overreach concerning ECT in children leaves one open-mouthed... This is ageism in reverse, and terribly unfair.' He asks: 'Are we denying children access to a treatment that is safe and effective in adults?'[6] This is expansionist rhetoric in a context where outcomes for electroshocked children have been no better than those for adults (see Youngsters).

The zealous pursuit of 'cure' is mirrored in the promotion of other technologies. For example, a company in Wales was recently granted approval by the US Food and Drug Administration to enter the USA market for 'device-based treatment of MDD [Major Depressive Disorder].' The Rapid2 stimulator uses a magnet instead of an electrical current to activate the brain. Magstim Company's 'stimulator' sends pulses of magnetic energy across the skull inducing electric current to flow and (according to the advertisements) activating neurons.[7]

The promotion of these more recent technologies is not limited to psychiatrists. Nick Davis is a lecturer in psychology at Swansea University. In a *Guardian* piece in May, 2015, he informs us that the magnetic pulses 'stimulate the left dorsolateral prefrontal cortex, the area of the brain associated with the regulation of mood.' This is claimed as a 'proven treatment option for those who have failed to respond to antidepressants or those unable to undergo medication.... This gives neuroscientists a way to reorganise (never 'rewire') small brain circuits.'

Davis's article is coy on the future of rTMS.

Although he says: 'The treatment certainly looks promising,' he points out: 'The uncertainties over the mechanisms of rTMS in MDD mean that neurologists will find it difficult to personalise treatment for an individual patient.'[8] As noted in Precision and Mervyn Peake, this is actually the case for all physical efforts to impact on metaphorical conditions.

The lure of magnetism shouldn't be regarded as a new phenomenon. In 1700, Michael Herwig published *The Art of Curing Sympathetically or Magnetically, Proved to be the Most True by its Theory and Practice.*[9] Herwig, however, uses the term magnetism as analogous to sympathy; now there is less profit to be made in sympathy.

A 2012 study had looked at forty-two US-based clinical TMS practice sites giving TMS to 307 outpatients inscribed with MDD. 'The primary outcome was change in the Clinician Global Impressions-Severity of Illness from baseline to end of acute phase. Secondary outcomes were change in continuous and categorical outcomes on self-report depression scales (9-Item Patient Health Questionnaire [PHQ-9], and Inventory of Depressive Symptoms-Self Report [IDS-SR])'.

The clinicians found remission (temporary improvement rate) in over a third of recipients while the remission rates self-reported via the PHQ-9 and IDS-SR were 28.7 and 26.5 per cent, respectively.[10] It is typical for clinicians to report better response rates than their patients (see Vested interest and Vaslav Nijinsky).

David Stein has also pointed out that: 'Validity and reliability of psychological tests are low, almost worthless ...'.[11] The authors, however, conclude: 'These data indicate that TMS is an effective treatment for those unable to benefit from initial antidepressant medication.'[12]

Zelda Fitzgerald

In April 1930, Zelda Fitzgerald (née Sayre) was admitted to a sanatorium in France where, after months of observation and treatment and a consultation with Eugen Bleuler, inventor of the term schizophrenia, she was inscribed as schizophrenic. Initially admitted to a hospital outside Paris, she was later moved to a clinic in Montreux, Switzerland.

The clinic primarily treated gastrointestinal ailments, and she was moved to a psychiatric facility in Prangins on the shores of Lake Geneva. She was released in September 1931. By February 1932, she had returned to living in a psychiatric clinic. Published later that year, she had written *Save Me the Waltz* in six weeks (Scott Fitzgerald had been working on *Tender is the Night* for five years).

Save Me the Waltz is a thinly disguised auto-biographical novel. The heroine, Alabama, 'had a strong sense of her own insignificance; of her life's slipping by ...'[13] Married to a successful, alcoholic philanderer, David, she embarks on a party-strewn tour of France, eventually spending time in a hospital close to death's door with an infection.

In 1936, Scott – already an alcoholic – placed his

novelist wife in the Highland Hospital in Asheville, North Carolina. He said that she claimed to be in direct contact with Christ, William the Conqueror, Mary Stuart and Apollo. She was released in March 1940.

Readmitted in 1943, on the night of March 10 1948, a fire broke out in the hospital kitchen. Zelda was locked into a room, awaiting electroshock. The fire moved through the dumbwaiter shaft, spreading onto every floor where the fire escapes were wooden. They too caught fire and nine women, including Zelda Fitzgerald, died.

Endnotes

Introduction

[1.] Harm, E. (1955). The origin and early history of electrotherapy and electroshock. *American Journal of Psychiatry, 111*, 933

[2.] Quoted in Palmer, R. L. (1981). The history of shock treatment. In R. L. Palmer (Ed.) *Electroconvulsive Therapy: An appraisal.* Oxford: Oxford University Press, p. 3.

[3.] Quoted in Harm op.cit.

[4.] http://www.bbc.co.uk/news/av/uk-england-coventry-warwickshire-36109638/shakespeare-is-man-who-pays-the-rent-dame-judi-dench

[5.] Frank Zappa cited in Watson, B. (1993). *The Negative Dialectics of Poodle Play.* London: Quartet Books p. 545 See also; Newnes, C. (2018). Towards coherence in teaching critical psy. In. C. Newnes and L. Golding (eds.) (2018). *Teaching Critical Psychology: International perspectives.* Abingdon: Routledge pp. 37-63 p.53

[6.] Rodgers, R. and Hammerstein II, O. (1959). *Do-Re-Mi* (song) New York: Hal Leonard Performing Arts Publishing Group

Assault and Antonin Artaud

[1.] Szasz, T.S. (2007). *Coercion as Cure: A Critical History of Psychiatry.* London: Transaction Publishers, p.10.

2. Stone, M. (1998). *Healing the Mind: A History of Psychiatry from Antiquity to the Present*. London: Pimlico, p.8.

3. Zilboorg, G. (1941). *A History of Medical Psychology*. New York: Norton.

4. Celsus (1953–1961). *De Medicina* (3 vols, trans. W.G. Spencer). Cambridge: Harvard University Press, pp.1–125. Quoted in Jackson S. W. (1986). *Melancholia and Depression*. New Haven, CT: Yale University Press. Jackson names hundreds of theorists and treatments, many aversive, the majority abandoned. See also; Valenstein, E. (1986). *Great and Desperate Cures: The Rise and Decline of Psychosurgery and Other Radical Treatments for Mental Illness*. New York: Basic Books.

5. Jones, Y. and Baldwin, S. (1992). ECT: Shock, lies and psychiatry. *Changes: An International Journal of Psychology and Psychotherapy, 10, 2,* 126–135.

6. Quoted in. Sontag, S. (Ed.) (1976). *Antonin Artaud: Selected Writings*. Berkeley, California: University of California Press. p. 530.

Bystanders and Bud Powell

1. Staub, E. (1989). *The Roots of Evil: The origins of genocide and other group violence*. New York: Cambridge University Press.

2. See, for example: Breggin, P. (1991). *Toxic Psychiatry: Why Therapy, Empathy and Love Must Replace the Drugs, Electroshock, and Biochemical Theories of the 'New Psychiatry.'* New York: St. Martin's Press; Breggin, P.R. (1998). Electroshock: Scientific, ethical, and political issues. *International*

Journal of Risk & Safety in Medicine, 11, 5 40.

3. Examples of clinical psychologists speaking out via publication include Baldwin, S. & Jones, Y. (1990). ECT, children and clinical psychologists: A shock to the system? *Clinical Psychology Forum, 25,* 2–4; Johnstone, L. (1999). Adverse psychological effects of ECT. *Journal of Mental Health, 8 (1)* 69–85; Johnstone, L. (2002). *Users and Abusers of Psychiatry: A critical look at psychiatric practice* (2nd ed.). London: Routledge; Newnes, C. (2016). *Inscription, Diagnosis and Deception in the Mental Health Industry: How Psy governs us all.* Basingstoke: Palgrave Macmillan; Newnes, C. (ed) (2015). *Children in Society: Politics, policies and interventions.* Ross on Wye: PCCS Books; Newnes, C. (2014). *Clinical Psychology: A critical examination.* Ross on Wye: PCCS Books; Newnes, C.D. (1991). ECT, the DCP and ME. *Clinical Psychology Forum, 36,* 20-24

4. Goldie, N. (1977). The division of labour among the mental health professions. In M. Stacey, M. Reid, C. Heath and R. Dingwall (eds) *Health and the Division of Labour.* London: Croom Helm, pp.141–161. 'Electroshock' doesn't appear in the index of *Clinical Psychology in Britain: Historical Perspectives* edited by Hall, J., Pilgrim, D., and Turpin, G. (2015). Leicester: British Psychological Society.

5. Editorial. (1904). *British Journal of Psychology, 1 (1)*

6. Beloff, J. (1973). *Psychological Sciences.* London: Staples.

7. Weber, M. (1948). Science as a Vocation. In S.H. Gerth and C. Wright Mills (eds), *From Max Weber.*

London: Routledge & Kegan Paul, quoted in Rose, N. (1989). *Governing the Soul: The Shaping of the Private Self.* London: Routledge., p.143.

8. http://wpedia.goo.ne.jp/enwiki/Journal_of_Clinical_ Psychology. Retrieved 4 January 2015.

9. Laing, R.D. (1985). *Wisdom, Madness and Folly: The making of a psychiatrist.* New York: McGraw-Hill. p.x Quoted in Szasz, T. (1987). *Insanity: The idea and its consequences.* New York: John Wiley & Sons p. 125

10. Breggin, P. (1985). The shame of my life. *AHP Perspective* (August-September): 9. Quoted in Szasz, T. (1987) *Insanity: The idea and its consequences.* New York: John Wiley & Sons p. 125

11. Stone, M.H. (1998). *Healing the Mind: A history of psychiatry from antiquity to the present.* London: Pimlico

12. Freedheim, D.K. (1992). *History of Psychotherapy: A century of change.* Washington: American Psychological Association

13. Johnstone, L. (2000). *Users and Abusers of Psychiatry: A critical look at psychiatric practice.* London: Routledge

14. Rowe, D. (1983). *Depression: The way out of your prison.* London: Routledge & Kegan Paul. p.175

15. Elwood, P. (2011). Lincolnshire's ECT Service http://www.lpft.nhs.uk/assets/files/InMind/InMind23 .pdf Retrieved December 17th 2017

16. Bill Evans quoted in. Paudras, F. (1998). *Dance of the Infidels: A Portrait of Bud Powell, (Trans: R. Monet)* New York: Da Capo Press. p.ix

17. Dyer, G. (2014). *But Beautiful: A Book About Jazz.*

New York: Farrar, Straus and Giroux.

18. Pullman, P. (2012). *Wail: The Life of Bud Powell*. New York: Peter Pullman LLC. http://www.wailthelifeofbudpowell.com/about-the-author/

Consent and Clementine Churchill

1. Valenstein, E. (1986). *Great and Desperate Cures: The Rise and Decline of Psychosurgery and Other Radical Treatments for Mental Illness*. New York: Basic Books.

2. Medawar, C. (1992). *Power and Dependence: Social Audit on the Safety of Medicines*. London: Social Audit Ltd. pp. 56-7

3. Berne, E. (1964). *Games People Play: The psychology of relationships*. New York: Grove Press

4. Fennell, P. (1996). *Treatment Without Consent: Law, psychiatry and the treatment of mentally disordered people since 1845*. London: Routledge

5. Fennel, op. cit. p.140

6. Bolam v Friern Hospital Management Committee [1957] 1 WLR 583 http://www.e-lawresources.co.uk/Bolam-v--Friern-Hospital-Management-Committee.php

7. Fennell, op. cit. p.6

8. Fennell, op. cit. p.172

9. http://www.cqc.org.uk/provider/RXT/inspection-summary#mhpsychintensive Retrieved 20th February, 2018

10. https://www.economist.com/blogs/gulliver/2015/01/air-safety Retrieved 20th February, 2018

11. Rose, D., Wykes, T., Bindman, J., Fleischmann, P. (2005). Information, consent and perceived coercion: patients' perspectives on electroconvulsive therapy. *British Journal of Psychiatry, 186*: 54-9

12. Leiknes,K.A., Jarosh-von Schweder, J., and Bjørg Høie, B. (2012). Contemporary use and practice of electroconvulsive therapy worldwide *Brain and Behaviour, 2* (3), 283–344.

13. http://psychiatrized.org/LeonardRoyFrank/ECTCons entForms/Electroschockconsentforms.pdf The APA Task Force form can be found on: http://psychiatrized.org/LeonardRoyFrank/ECTConse ntForms/ExamplesofConsentForms.pdf Retrieved 20th February, 2018

14. Baldwin, S. and Oxlad, M. (1996). Multiple case sampling of ECT administration to 217 minors. *Journal of Mental Health, 5,* (5), 451-63

15. Baldwin, S. and Jones, Y. (1990). ECT and children. *Changes: An International Journal of Psychology and Psychotherapy, 8,* 1, 30-39 p.34

16. Pilgrim, D. (1990). When the talking has to stop. An interview with Jeffrey Masson. *Changes: An International Journal of Psychology and Psychotherapy, 8,* 1, 40-48 p.43

17. Post, F. (1994). Creativity and psychopathology: A study of 291 world-famous men. *British Journal of Psychiatry, 165,* 22–34.

18. https://www.facebook.com/PsychVictims/posts/634 820743367162 Retrieved 20th February, 2018

Death-making and David Reville

1. Wolfensberger, W. (1987). *The New Genocide of Handicapped and Afflicted People*. New York: University of Syracuse

2. Foucault, M. (1976). *The Birth of the Clinic. An archaeology of medical perception*. London: Tavistock

3. Gruenberg, E. (1966). *Evaluating the Effectiveness of Community Mental Health Services*. New York: Milbank Publishers.

4. Weindling, P. (1989). *Health, Race and German Politics between National Unification and Nazism 1870-1945* Cambridge: Cambridge University Press

6. Lifton, R. J. (1988). *The Nazi Doctors: Medical killing and the psychology of genocide*. London: Little Brown Book Group

7. Proctor, R.N. (1988). *Racial Hygiene: Medicine under the Nazis*. Cambridge, MA.: Harvard University Press Quoted in. Bentall, R.P. (2003). *Madness Explained: Psychosis and Human Nature*. London: Penguin - Allen Lane p.498

8. Weindling op.cit. p 543

9. Lehmann, P. (2017). Irreconcilable Memory Culture in Psychiatry: Congratulations on Dorothea Buck's 100th Birthday *The Journal of Critical Psychology, Counselling and Psychotherapy 17, 2*. 112-120 p.113

10. Cattell, R.B. (1972). *A New Morality from Science: Beyondism*. New York: Pergamon Press, p.220.

11. See; http://www.mindfreedom.org/who-we-are/who-we-are

293

Evidence and Electrocution

1. Newnes, C. D. (1991). ECT, the DCP and ME. *Clinical Psychology Forum, 36*, 20–4.

2. Eranti, S. & McLoughlin, D. M. (2003). Electroconvulsive therapy – state of the art. *British Journal of Psychiatry, 182*, 8–9.

3. *Ibid.*

4. Bickerton, D., Worrall, A. & Chaplin, R. (2009). Trends in the administration of electroconvulsive therapy in England. *The Psychiatrist, 33*, 61–63

5. Read, J. Harrop, C. Geekie, J. and Renton, J. (2017). An audit of ECT in England 2011–2015: Usage, demographics, and adherence to guidelines and legislation *Psychology and Psychotherapy: Theory, Research and Practice* See: https//www.google.co.uk/search?q=An+audit+of+ECT +in+England+2011%E2%80%932015%3A+Usage%2C +demographics%2C+and+adherence+to+guidelines+a nd+legislation&oqs=chrome..69i57j69i64.2424j0j8&so urceid=chrome&ie=UTF-8 Retrieved 21st December, 2017

6. Piper, R. (2018). Fear and loathing in the education system. In. C. Newnes and L. Golding (eds.) *Teaching Critical Psychology: International perspectives* London: Routledge

7. Avery, D. and Winokur, G. (1976). Mortality in depressed patients treated with ECT and antidepressants. *Archives of General Psychiatry, 33*, 1029-1037

8. Breggin, P.R. (1997). *Brain Disabling Treatments in Psychiatry: Drugs, electroshock and the role of the*

FDA. New York: Springer Publishing Company p.136

9. Newnes, C. (2014). *Clinical Psychology: A critical examination*. Monmouth: PCCS Books

10. Palis, D.J. and Stoffelmayr, B.E. (1973). Social attitudes and treatment among psychiatrists. *British Journal of Medical Psychology, 46,* 75-81 In. Jones, Y. and Baldwin, S. (1992). ECT: Shock, lies and psychiatry. *Changes: An International Journal of Psychology and Psychotherapy, 10, 2,* 126-135 p.131

11. Frank, L.R. (1990). Electroshock: Death, brain damage, memory loss and brainwashing. *The Journal of Mind and Behaviour: An interdisciplinary journal, Summer/Autumn, 11, (3 and 4),* 489-512 p.505 Dozens of links to Frank's work are available on http://psychiatrized.org/LeonardRoyFrank/FromTheF ilesOfLeonardRoyFrank.htm

12. McClelland, R.J., Fenton, G.W., and Rutherford, W. (1994). The postconcussional syndrome revisited. *Journal of the Royal Society of Medicine, 87,* 507-510 Cited in Breggin (1997). op. cit. pp140-141

13. Friedberg, (1977). Shock treatment, brain damage and memory loss: A neurological perspective. *American Journal of Psychiatry, 134,* 1010-1014

14. Babayan, E. (1985). *The Structure of Psychiatry in the Soviet Union*. New York: International Universities Press. p.37

15. Breggin, op.cit. p.148

16. Breggin, *ibid* p.146

17. Impastato, D.J. (1957, July). Prevention of fatalities in electroshock therapy. *Diseases of the Nervous System, 18*(7), (sect.2), 34-74

18. Yildiz, A., Ruiz, P., and Nemeroff, C.B. (2015). *The Bipolar Book: History, Neurobiology and Treatment* Oxford: Oxford University

19. Mukherjee, S., Sackheim, H.A., and Schnur, D.B. (1994). Electroconvulsive therapy of acute manic episodes: A review of 50 years' experience. *The American Journal of Psychiatry, 151,* (2), 169-176. American Psychiatric Association. (2001). *The practice of ECT: Recommendations for treatment, training and privileging (*2nd. ed.) Washington DC: American Psychiatric Press. National Institute for Clinical Excellence. (2003). *Guidance on the use of electroconvulsive therapy.* London: National Institute for Clinical Excellence

20. McNichol, T. (2006). *AC/DC: The savage tale of the First Standards war.* NY: Jossey-Bass

21. Cerletti U., & Bini L. (1938). L'Elettroshock. *Archivio Generale di Neurologia, Psichiatria e Psicoanalisi, 19*: 266-268.

22. Endler, N.S. (1988). The Origins of Electroconvulsive Therapy (ECT) *Convulsive Therapy 4(1)* 5-23

23. Passione, R. (2008). 'Non solo l'elettroshock: Ugo Cerletti e il rinnovamento della Psichiatria italiana. In Marco Piccolino (ed.), *Neuroscienze Controverse: Da Aristotele alla moderna scienza del linguaggio.* Torino: Bollati Boringhieri. p.258. See also; Passione, R. (2007). *Il Romanzo dell'elettroshock* Reggio Emilia: Aliberti pp. 68–9.

24. Accornero, F. (1970). Testimonianza oculare sulla scoperta dell'elettroshock, *Pagine di storia della medicina, 14,* 2, 39-49.

25. Aruta, A. (2011). Shocking Waves at the Museum: The Bini–Cerletti Electro-shock Apparatus *Medical History 55(3):* 407–412.

26. *Ibid.* p. 407

27. https://www.ectron.co.uk/ Accessed 5th March, 2018

28. http://www.oprah.com/spirit/beyond-prozac-depression-treatment-breakthroughs Retrieved Jan 17 2018.

Fits and Frances Farmer

1. For a patient-centred account of the immediate effects of electroshock (the viewer is positioned as the recipient via the camera shots), see *We're Not Mad, We're Angry.* https://www.youtube.com/watch?v=qD36m1mveoY.

2. http://ectstatistics.wordpress.com/2013/05/20/75-years-of-electroconvulsivetherapy/. Retrieved 30 May 2013.

3. Breggin, P. (1991). *Toxic Psychiatry: Why Therapy, Empathy and Love Must Replace the Drugs, Electroshock, and Biochemical Theories of the 'New Psychiatry.'* New York: St. Martin's Press.

4. Breggin, P.R. (1998). Electroshock: Scientific, ethical, and political issues. *International Journal of Risk & Safety in Medicine, 11*, 5–40.

5. Weiner, R.D. (1980). The persistence of ECT induced changes in the electroencephalogram. *Journal of Mental Disease, 168*, 224–228.

6. Symonds, C.P. (1966). Disorders of memory. *Brain, 89*, 625–640.

7. See Frank, L.R.(1990). Electroshock: Death, brain

damage, memory loss and brainwashing. *Journal of Mind and Behaviour, II,* 3–4, 489–512.

8. McClelland, R.J. (1988), Psychosocial sequaelae of head injury: An anatomy of a relationship. *British Journal of Psychiatry, 153,* 141–146.

9. Electroconvulsive Therapy: Schizophrenia https://www.youtube.com/watch?v=0Npc7IThVqc Retrieved; 14th February, 2018

10. Wilcox, P.H. (1946). Brain facilitation, not brain destruction, the aim in electroshock therapy. *Diseases of the Nervous System, 7,* 201-204, and Wilcox, P.H. (1972). Electrostimulation for promoting brain reorganization. *Diseases of the Nervous System, 33,* 326-327

11. Cameron, D. (1994). ECT: Sham statistics, the myth of convulsive therapy, and the case for consumer misinformation. *The Journal of Mind and Behaviour, 15, (2)* 177-198 p. 183

12. Ebaugh, F., Barnacle, C., and Neuberger, K. (1943). Fatalities following electroconvulsive therapy. *Archives of Neurological Psychiatry, 49,* 107-117

13. Brody, M.P. (1944). Prolonged memory deficits following electrotherapy. *Journal of Mental Science, 90,* 777-779

14. Saltzman, L. (1947). An evaluation of shock therapy. *American Journal of Psychiatry, 103,* 676

15. https://www.stanfordbrainstorm.com/ Retrieved 10th January 2018

16. Neher, A. (1962). A physiological explanation of unusual behaviour in ceremonies involving drums. *Human Biology, 34,* 151-160 Cited in Fuller Torrey, E.

(1986). *Witchdoctors and Psychiatrists: The common roots of psychotherapy and its future* Northvale, NJ.: Aronson.

[17.] Jilek, W.G. (1982). Altered states of consciousness in North American Indian ceremonials. *Ethos, 10,* 326-343 Cited in Fuller Torrey, op.cit.

[18.] Fuller Torrey, E. (1986). *Witchdoctors and Psychiatrists: The common roots of psychotherapy and its future* Northvale, NJ.: Aronson. p.94

[19.] Harris, M. and Landis, CL (1997). *Sexual Abuse in the Lives of Women Diagnosed with Serious Mental Illness (New Directions in Therapeutic Intervention)* London: Routledge p.146

Governmentality and Gene Tierney

[1.] Bentham, J. (1843). *The Works of Jeremy Bentham, vol. 4 (Panopticon, Constitution, Colonies, Codification)* p.39
http://oll.libertyfund.org/titles/bentham-the-works-of-jeremy-bentham-vol-4#lf0872-04_head_004
Retrieved March 19th 2017

[2.] Foucault, M. (1979). On governmentality. *Ideology and Consciousness, 6,* 5–22, p.20. 2.

[3.] Rose, N. (1989). *Governing the Soul: The Shaping of the Private Self.* London: Routledge. p.142.

[4.] *Ibid.* See Plate 1, p.143.

[5.] *Ibid.* p.144

[6.] Pilgrim, D. and Treacher, A. (1992). *Clinical Psychology Observed.* London: Routledge, p.190.

[7.] Rejali, D. (2007). *Torture and Democracy.* Princeton: Princeton University Press. p. 4. Cited in. Pick, A.

(2017). Sparks would fly. In. Lundblad, M. (ed.) *Animalities: Literary and Cultural Studies Beyond the Human.* Edinburgh: Edinburgh University Press. pp. 104-126

8. Pick, A. (2017). Sparks would fly. In. Lundblad, M. (ed.) *Animalities: Literary and Cultural Studies Beyond the Human.* Edinburgh: Edinburgh University Press. pp. 104-126 p.104

9. Plath, S. (1963). *The Bell Jar* London: Faber and Faber p.138

10. Phillips, P. (1938). *Annual Report to the Governors of Bethlem Royal Hospital. Physician Superintendent's Report.* HMSO: London p.8

11. Plath op.cit. p.203

History and Hemingway

1. Harm, E. (1955). The origin and early history of electrotherapy and electroshock. *American Journal of Psychiatry, 111,* 933.

2. Quoted in Palmer, R. L. (1981). The history of shock treatment. In R. L. Palmer (Ed.). *Electroconvulsive Therapy: An appraisal.* Oxford: Oxford University Press, p. 3.

3. Quoted in Harm (1955). See note 1.

4. Beard, G.M. and Rothwell, A.D. (1892). *Medical and Surgical Uses of Electricity* (8th edn). New York: Wm. Wood. See Valenstein, op. cit., p.24.

5. Cushman, P. (1992). Psychotherapy to 1992: A historically situated interpretation. In D.K. Freedheim (ed.) *History of Psychotherapy: A Century of Change.* Washington, DC: American Psychological Association,

pp. 21–64

6. Teilleux, M. (1859). De l'Application de l'Electricity au Traitement d'Alienation Mentale *Annales Medico-Psychologique*

7. Neuth, A.H. (1884). The Value of Electricity in the Treatment of Insanity. *The British Journal of Psychiatry Oct 1884, 30 (131)* 354-359

8. http://www.dailymail.co.uk/news/article-2462653/Haunting-images-abandoned-mental-hospital-patients-subject-cruel-treatments.html#ixzz51VQiLTAQ Retrieved. December 17th 2017

9. Murray, R.M. and Turner, T.H. (1990). *Lectures on the History of Psychiatry: The Squib series*. London: Gaskell p.108

10. Stone, M. (1998). *Healing the Mind: A history of psychiatry from antiquity to the present*. London: Pimlico, p. 8.

11. Attempts to link madness to genuine organic pathology (other than that caused by medication) continue. A study from Chicago's Northwestern University screened the blood of teenagers for 26 markers found to be present in those with depression (according to animal studies). *The Daily Telegraph*, explicitly reports, 'Finding a biological sign of depression also confirms that the condition is a disease.' Smith, R. (2014). Chemical link to teenagers with depression. *The Daily Telegraph,* September 15, p. 13.

12. Valenstein, E. (1986). *Great and Desperate Cures: The Rise and Decline of Psychosurgery and Other*

Radical Treatments for Mental Illness. New York: Basic Books. Meduna's claims for success have subsequently been challenged and the overall remission rate reduced. See Baran, B., Bitter, I., Ungvari, G.S. and Gazdag, G. (2012). The birth of convulsive therapy revisited: A reappraisal of László Meduna's first cohort of patients. *Journal of Affective Disorders, 136, 3,* 1179–1182. PubMed Abstract. The FDA withdrew its license for metrazol in 1982.

[13.] Lindow, V. (1993). 'Thinking about ECT.' Shropshire Institute of Mental Health seminar series 'Alternatives to Psychiatry': Shropshire Mental Health Authority. December 1993. See also; Lindow, V. (1999). Survivor controlled alternatives to psychiatric services. In C. Newnes, G. Holmes and C. Dunn (eds.), *This Is Madness: A Critical Look at Psychiatry and the Future of Mental Health Services.* Ross-on-Wye: PCCS Books. pp.211–226.

[14.] Valenstein, E. op. cit. p.51

[15.] Shorter, E. (1997), *A History of Psychiatry: From the era of the asylum to the age of Prozac.* Chichester: John Wiley & Sons p.220

[16.] *Ibid.* p.221

[17.] In 1988, Hotchner and Paul Newman co-founded, in Ashford, Connecticut, the Hole in the Wall Gang Camp, a residential summer camp and year-round centre for seriously ill children. By 2016, as part of the SeriousFun Children's Network, there were 30 camps and programmes serving over 130,000 children and families around the world.

[18.] Hotchner, A.E. (1967). *Papa Hemingway* New York:

Bantam. p.308 Cited in. Frank, L.R. (1990). Electroshock: Death, brain damage, memory loss and brainwashing. *The Journal of Mind and Behaviour: An interdisciplinary journal, Summer/Autumn, 11, (3 and 4),* 489-512 p.508

Inscription and Insulin coma

[1.]The Psy complex is Rose's term for the financial/professional/linguistic disciplinary apparatus governing us all. See: Rose, N. (1989). *Governing the Soul: The Shaping of the Private Self.* London: Routledge.

[2.] Warner, S. (1996). The drive towards numbers for credible research in clinical psychology. *Changes: An International Journal of Psychology and Psychotherapy, 14, 3,* 187–191.

[3.] Healey, A. (2017). Northampton require shock therapy. *The Daily Telegraph,* December 22nd.

[4.] Marr, A. (2007). *A History of Modern Britain.* London: Macmillan. p. 262

[5.] Leo, J. (1985). Battling over masochism. TIME, Dec. 2, 76

[6.] Haslam, J. (1810). *Illustrations of Madness, Exhibiting a Singular Case of Insanity, and a No Less Remarkable Difference of Medical Opinion: Developing the Nature of Assailment, and the Manner of Working Events; with a Description of the Tortures Experienced by Bomb-Bursting, Lobster-Cracking and Lengthening the Brain, Embellished with a Curious Plate.* London: Rivingtons, Robinsons, Callow, Murray & Greenland.

7. Porter, R. (1988). *Illustrations of Madness*. London: Routledge. Introduction, p.xxviii.

8. Haslam, op. cit., p.15.

9. Berrios, G.E. (1996). *The History of Mental Symptoms: Descriptive Psychopathology Since the Nineteenth Century*. Cambridge: Cambridge University Press, p.34.

10. Hill, C.G. (1907). quoted in Grob, G.N. (1991) Origins of DSM-I: A study in appearance and reality. *American Journal of Psychiatry, 148, 4*, 421–431.

11. Katz, J. (1983). Cited in Szasz, T. (1987). *Insanity: The idea and its consequences*. Chichester: John Wiley & Sons, p. 145.

12. Retrieved 30th May 2013 from http://ectstatistics.wordpress.com/2013/03/18/ectin-greece-and-turkey/

13. See also; Piper, R. (2018). Fear and loathing in the education system. In. C. Newnes and L. Golding (eds.) *Teaching Critical Psychology: International perspectives*. London: Routledge pp. 82-99

14. Manfred Sakel (1900–1957) claimed direct lineal descent from Moses Maimonides, twelfth-century physician, rabbi and philosopher. Wortis, J. (1958/9). In Memoriam. Manfred Sakel MD, 1900–1957. *American Journal of Psychiatry, 115*, 287–288.

15. Sakel, M. (1954). The classical shock treatment: A reappraisal. *Journal of Clinical and Experimental Psychopathology and Quarterly Review of Psychiatry and Neurology, 15, 3,* 262.

16. Sakel later suggested that insulin coma worked by 'causing an intensification of the tonus of the

parasympathetic end of the autonomic nervous system, by blockading the nerve cell, and by strengthening the anabolic force which induces the restoration of the normal function of the nerve cell and the recovery of the patient.' Sakel, M.J. (1956). The classical Sakel shock treatment: a reappraisal. In. A. M. Sackler, M.D. Sackler, R.R. Sackler, and F. Marti-Ibanez. (eds.) *The great physiodynamic therapies in psychiatry: an historical reappraisal.* Hoeber-Harper: New York: 13-75

[17.] Sandison, R. (2001). *A Century of Psychiatry, Psychotherapy and Group Analysis: A Search for Integration.* London: Jessica Kingsley Publishers, p.21.

[18.] Dax, E.C. (1947). *Modern Mental Treatment: a handbook for nurses.* London: Faber pp.13-14

[19.] Bourne, H. (1953). The insulin myth. *Lancet. Ii. 265 (6798):* 964–8

[20.] Gittens, D. (1998). *Narratives of Severalls Hospital, 1913-1977.* Oxford: Oxford University Press 197-199

[21.] Mayer-Gross, W., Slater, E. and Roth, M. (1960). *Clinical Psychiatry* (2nd edn). London: Cassell, p.245. Quoted in Valenstein, E. (1986). *Great and Desperate Cures: The Rise and Decline of Psychosurgery and Other Radical Treatments for Mental Illness.* New York: Basic Books. p.59

[22.] Stone, M.H. (1998). *Healing the Mind: A History of Psychiatry from Antiquity to the Present.* London: Pimlico.

[23.] Farber, S. (1993). From victim to revolutionary: An interview with Leonard Frank. In S. Farber (ed.) *Madness, Heresy and the Rumour of Angels: The*

Revolt Against the Mental Health System. Chicago and La Salle, Illinois: Open Court, pp.190–240, p.195.

Justification and Janet Frame

[1.]For a discussion of the different types of social power see; Goldie, N. (1977). The division of labour among the mental health professions. In M. Stacey, M. Reid, C. Heath and R. Dingwall (eds.) *Health and the Division of Labour*. London: Croom Helm, pp.141–161.

[2.] Donnelly, L. (2017). Half of English adults now on medication. *The Daily Telegraph*. Thursday, 14th December. p.6

[3.] Rose, N. (1989). *Governing the Soul: The Shaping of the Private Self*. London: Routledge.

[4.] Levine, B. (2014). 10 Ways Mental Health Professionals Increase Misery in Suffering People. *The Journal of Critical Psychology, Counselling and Psychotherapy, 14, (1),* 23-29

[5.]This stance is increasingly taken by those accused of assault (soccer players in night-clubs) and driving offences, especially those involving alcohol (anyone who happens to be taking anti-depressants).

[6.] Breggin, P.R. (1997). *Brain Disabling Treatments in Psychiatry: Drugs, electroshock and the role of the FDA*. New York: Springer Publishing Company   See also; Sapin, P. (Producer) (1994). *Welcome to Happy Valley [TV documentary]*. UK: Everyman BBC Production.

https://www.youtube.com/watch?v=vM3k-ghKerI

[7.] American Psychiatric Association (1978). *Electroconvulsive Therapy* Task Force Report 14.

Washington D.C.: American Psychiatric Association p. 8.

[8.] Viscott, D. (1972). *The Making of a Psychiatrist*. Greenwich, Connecticut: Faucett. p. 356 Cited in. Frank, L. (1990). Electroshock: Death, brain damage, memory loss and brainwashing. *The Journal of Mind and Behaviour, 11, 4,* 243-266

[9.] Frank op.cit. p. 248

[10.]https://en.wikipedia.org/wiki/Janet_Frame Retrieved January 1st 2018

[11.] Frame, J. (1982). *To the Is-Land* (Autobiography 1) and Frame, J. (1984). *An Angel at My Table* (Autobiography 2). Both; New York: Braziller. Frame, J. (1984). *The Envoy From Mirror City* (Autobiography). Auckland: Century Hutchinson.

Killing with kindness and Kitty Dukakis

[1.] Vonnegut, Jr., K. (1968). *Mother Night*. London: Jonathan Cape. Quoted in. Newnes, C. (1993). After Vonnegut. *Changes: An International Journal of Psychology and Psychotherapy, 11, 4,* 293-302

[2.] Breggin, P. (1991). *Toxic Psychiatry. Why therapy, empathy, and love must replace the drugs, electroshock, and biochemical theories of the 'new psychiatry.'* London: Harper Collins

[3.] An increasing factor in referral to specialist health services is the GP:patient ratio. Kindly - usually male - physicians who spent hours with patients offering advice may have existed before the days when television created iconic myths such as Dr Kildare but, for over forty years the claim that GPs don't have the time to talk to patients has gathered momentum. Whether conversations with GPs are better than chats with neighbours is a moot point; the expectancy on both sides that the GP must *do* something as quickly as possible will result in a prescription or referral, often within minutes.

4. Szasz, T. (1974). *The Myth of Mental Illness: Foundations of a theory of personal conduct*. (Revised edition, first published 1961) New York: Harper Collins.

5. http://www.ect.org/resources/california.html Retrieved 30th May 2013

6. Reid, W. H., Keller, S., Leatherman, M. & Mason, M. (1998). ECT in Texas: 19 months of mandatory reporting. *Journal of Clinical Psychiatry, 59* (1), 8–13, p. 13.

7. Scull, A. (1990). Desperate remedies: A Gothic tale of madness and modern medicine. In. R.M. Murray and T.H. Turner (eds.) *Lectures on the History of Psychiatry: The Squibb Series*. London: Gaskell/Royal College of Psychiatrists pp.144-169 p.167

8. Seelye, K.Q. (2017). Beneficiary of Electroshock Therapy Emerges as Its Leading Evangelist. *New York Times, A13* January 1st 2017

9. https://files.acrobat.com/a/preview/8068ec6b-c78c-4bad-a616-7d8ce1690ee0 Retrieved 5th January 2018

Law and Lou Reed

1. Kate Millet interview in O'Hagan, M. (1993). *Stopovers on My Way Home from Mars: a journey into the psychiatric survivor movement in the USA, Britain and the Netherlands*. London: Survivors Speak

Out. O'Hagan's travel was sponsored by the Winston Churchill Memorial Trust, an organization that supports exploration of innovatory practice and, perhaps, owes its 1965 origins to Clementine. See; Consent and Clementine Churchill https://www.thersa.org/fellowship/fellowship-news/fellowship-news/winston-churchill-memorial-2017-travel-scholarships?gclid=CjwKCAiArOnUBRBJEiwAXorG_Q VUWbrZinWYa2c_h81jUrJo2te7YxrtPORyu2JHELRD v89mQyvN5RoCR-IQAvD_BwE Accessed 3[d] Mar 2018.

2. Eli Lilly was a large contributor to the senatorial campaigns of Dan Quayle, instrumental in passing legislation described as a Lilly spokesman as the, '... most important drug measure before Congress at that time.' Quoted in Breggin, P. (1991). *Toxic Psychiatry: Why therapy, empathy and love must replace the drugs, electroshock and biochemical theories of the 'new psychiatry.'* New York: St. Martin's Press. Footnote, p. 151

3. Cohen, J. (Ed.) (1975). *The Essential Lenny Bruce: His original unexpurgated satirical routines.* St. Albans: Panther Books. p.75

4. http://digital.nhs.uk/catalogue/PUB22571 Retrieved 5th March, 2018

5. Hervey, N. (1985). A slavish bowing down: the Lunacy Commission and the psychiatric profession. In. W.F. Bynum, R. Porter and M. Shepherd (eds.) *The Anatomy of Madness Vol. II: Institutions and society.* London: Tavistock Publications pp.98-131 p.98

6. *Ibid.* p.101

7. Mackenzie, C. (1992). *Psychiatry for the Rich: A history of Ticehurst private asylum.* London: Routledge

8. Clark, M.J. (1993). Law, liberty and psychiatry in Victorian Britain; an historical survey and commentary, c.1840 – c.1890. In. de Goie, L. and Vijselaar, J. (eds.) *Proceedings: 1st European Congress on the History of Psychiatry and Mental Health Care.* Rotterdam: Erasmus Publishing pp.188-193

9. Kessler, M. and Albee, G. (1975). Primary prevention. *Annual Review of Psychology, 30,* 557-591 Quoted in Newnes, C.D. (1990). Counselling and Primary Prevention. *Counselling Psychology Quarterly 3,* 2, 205-210 p.205

10. Weindling, P. (1989). *Health, Race and German Politics between National Unification and Nazism 1870-1945* Cambridge: Cambridge University Press p.546

11. Barham, P. (1992). *Closing the Asylum: The mental patient in modern society.* London: Penguin. p. 141

12. Basaglia, F. (1977). *Libération* January

13. Illich, I. (1978). *The Right to Useful Unemployment and its Professional Enemies.* London: Marion Boyars Publishers Limited

14. Foucault, M. (1976). *The Birth of the Clinic. An archaeology of medical perception.* London: Tavistock

15. Busfield, J. (1986). *Managing Madness: Changing ideas and practice.* London: Unwin Hyman

16. Fennell, P. (1996). *Treatment Without Consent: Law, psychiatry and the treatment of mentally disordered people since 1845.* London: Routledge p.

175-6

17. Rosen, J. (1953). *Direct Analysis: Selected papers.* New York: Grune & Stratton.

18. Masson, J. (1989). *Against Therapy.* London: William Collins Sons & Co. Ltd Footnote 1, p.165

19. Amended Citation October 19th 1982 (File Nos. 77-ME-1221 and 81-ME-889). Quoted in Masson, op. cit. p. 186

20. Masson, op. cit. p.210

21. http://www.bookbuzzr.com/books/4376/THE-INSANITY-WARS Accessed 4 March, 2018.

22. In. Baldwin, S. and Jones, Y. (1992). ECT: shock, lies and psychiatry. *Changes: An International Journal of Psychology and Psychotherapy, 10,* 2, 126-135 p.132

23. Breggin, P. (1991). *Toxic Psychiatry: Why therapy, empathy and love must replace the drugs, electroshock and biochemical theories of the 'new psychiatry.'* New York: St. Martin's Press. p.213

24. Dörner, K. and Plog, U. (1992). *Irren ist menschlich Lehrbuch der Psychiatrie/Psychotherapie* (7th Edition) Bonn: Psychiatrieverlag Quoted in. Lehmann, P. (1994). 'Progressive' psychiatry. *International Journal of Psychology and Psychotherapy, 12,* 1, 37-49 p.43

25. http://caselaw.findlaw.com/tx-court-of-appeals/1546616.html Retrieved January, 11th 2017

26. ectstatistics (2017) *ECT at Cypress Creek Hospital, Houston, Texas.* Posted on December 27 2017 by ectstatistics. Retrieved January 11 2017

27. Pegler, J. (2004). Out of the darkness. *21st Century Asylums? Essays about low secure hospitals in the field of learning disabilities.* pp. 44-50 p.46

28. Lorandos, D., and Campbell, T.W. (2005). *Benchbook in the Behavioral Sciences.* Durham, NC: Carolina Academic Press and Mischel, W. (1996). *Personality and Assessment.* Mahwah, NJ: Lawrence Erlbaum Associates.

29. Stein, D. B. (2012). *The Psychology Industry under a Microscope!* Plymouth, UK: University Press of America Inc.

30. Law Report (2017) Assessing the divisibility of a psychiatric injury. Court of Appeal, September 27th 2017. Judgement July 31 2017. [2017] EWCA Civ 1188 *The Times,* Wednesday, September, 27 2017 p. 59

31. Psychiatric inpatient comment to Shelton Patients' Council. In. Newnes, C. (2001). Speaking out. *Ethical Human Sciences and Services, 3,* 1, 53-60 p.57

32. Blom-Cooper, l. (1995). *Report of the committee of inquiry into Ashworth Special Hospital.* London: The Stationary Office, and Fallon, P., Bluglass, R., Edwards, B. & Daniels, G. (1999). *Report of the committee of inquiry into the personality disorder unit Ashworth Special Hospital.* London: The Stationary Office

33. Kellner, C.H. (July 5, 2011). The FDA Advisory Panel on the Reclassification of ECT Devices: *Unjustified Ambivalence. Psych Times, Vol 28,* 7 https://www.webcitation.org/6BgaDd9Hc?url=http://www.psychiatrictimes.com/electroconvulsive-therapy/content/article/10168/1897020

34. Bynum, W.F. (1985). The nervous patient in eighteenth- and nineteenth-century Britain: the psychiatric origins of British neurology. In. W.F.Bynum, R.Porter, and M.Shepherd (eds.) *The*

Anatomy of Madness: Essays in the history of psychiatry. Volume I: People and ideas. London: Tavistock pp. 89-102 p.92

35. National Association of State Mental Health Program Directors (2006, October). Morbidity and Mortality in People with Serious Mental Illness. Available on the Internet at http://psychrights.org/Articles/2006NASMHPDonEarlyDeath.pdf

36. Gottstein, J. (2018). Psychiatry and the Law: The Law Project for Psychiatric Rights' public education approach. In C. Newnes and L.Golding (eds.) *Teaching Critical psychology: International perspectives.* London: Routledge pp. 170-194

37. Newnes, C. (2009). Are we all mad? *Psychotherapy Section Review, 47,* 18-22

38. Fergusson, G. (Chair); et al. (2009). 'The Scottish ECT Accreditation Network (SEÁN) Annual Report 2009' (PDF). Scottish ECT Accreditation Network. Retrieved 6th March, 2018

39. Lehmann, P. (2015). Securing human rights in the psychiatric field by utilizing advance directives. *Journal of Critical Psychology, Counselling and Psychotherapy, 15* (1) 1–10.

40. McCourt, J. (2001). User-friendly research in clinical psychology. *The Psychologist, 14,* 6, 296-7.

41. Szasz, T. (1990). Law and psychiatry: The problems that will not go away. *The Journal of Mind and Behaviour, 4,* 311-317 p.311.

42. Szasz, T. (1977). *Psychiatric Slavery.* Syracuse, NY: Syracuse University Press.

43. *O'Connor v. Donaldson,* 422 US 563 (1975).

44. Kelley, J.L. (1996). *Psychiatric Malpractice: Stories of patients, psychiatrists, and the law*. New Brunswick, NJ: Rutgers University Press p.123

45. Guralnick, P. (2015). *Sam Phillips: The man who invented Rock 'n' Roll*. New York: Little, Brown.

Marketing and the movies

1. Drabble, M. (2000). *The Oxford Companion to English Literature*. 6th Edition. Oxford: Oxford University Press. p.147

2. https://en.wikisource.org/wiki/A_Blighted_Life Retrieved. 20 January 2018

3. Donnelly, L. (2018). Call for more anxiety drugs *Daily Telegraph 22nd February* pp.1-2

4. Jones, Y. and Baldwin, S. (1992). ECT: Shock, lies and psychiatry. *Changes: An International Journal of Psychology and Psychotherapy, 10, 2,* 126–135, p.134.

5. Mangold, J. (Director) (2010). *Knight and Day* [film]. New York: 20th Century Fox.

6. Ghaziuddin, N., Kaza, M., Ghazi, N., King, C., Walter, G. & Rey, J. M. (2001). Electroconvulsive therapy for minors: Experiences and attitudes of child psychiatrists and psychologists. *Journal of Electroconvulsive Therapy, 17,* 109–117.

7. Ross, C. A. (2006). The Sham ECT Literature: Implications for consent to ECT. *Ethical Human Psychology and Psychiatry, 8 (1)* 17–28, p. 26.

8. Royal College of Psychiatrists *Information on ECT* http://www.rcpsych.ac.uk/healthadvice/treatmentswel lbeing/ect.aspx Retrieved, 16 March, 2015.

9. http://www.rcpsych.ac.uk/mentalhealthinformation/t

herapies/electroconvulsivetherapy,ect.aspx   Retrieved 28 February, 2018.

10. Enns, M. W. & Reiss, J. P. (2015). Electroconvulsive therapy (Canadian Psychiatric Association Position Paper, published 16 March 2015). Available at https://ww1.cpaapc.org/Publications/Position_Papers /Therapy.asp Retrieved 28th February, 2018.

11. Ghaziuddin, N. & Walter, G. (eds.) (2013). *Electroconvulsive Therapy in Children and Adolescents.* Oxford: Oxford University Press.

12. Kirov, G. (2017). Electroconvulsive therapy does work – and it can be miraculous http://www.independent.co.uk/news/health/electroco nvulsive-therapy-does-work-and-it-can-be-miraculous-a7695391.html Retrieved, 27 February, 2018.

13. https://www.youtube.com/watch?v=3h2vqk_woa8

14. Rosenhan, D. (1973). On being sane in insane places. *Science. 179 (4070):* 250–258/

15. http:www.smh.com.au/entertainment/movies/madn ess-at-the-movies-why-hollywood-went-crazy-for-freud-20150328-1m928k.html Retrieved 14th January, 2018.

16. See Scull, A. (2015). *Madness in Civilisation: A cultural history of insanity, from the Bible to Freud, from the madhouse to modern medicine.* Princeton, NJ: Princeton University Press.

17. Breggin, P.R. (1998). Electroshock: Scientific, ethical and political issues. *International Journal of Risk & Safety in Medicine, 11,* 5-40.

18. Faith, K. (1993). *Unruly Women: The politics of confinement & resistance.* Vancouver: Press Gang

Publishers

19. Rapley, M. (2018). Sigmund and Michel, Alain and Mary Go Shopping: The commodification of misery. *Journal of Critical Psychology, Counselling and Psychotherapy, 17, 1*

20. Moynihan, R. Heath, I. & Henry, D. (2002). Selling sickness: the pharmaceutical industry and disease mongering. *British Medical Journal, 324,* (7342), 886–91.

Normality and novels

1. Foucault, M. (1979). *Discipline and Punish.* Harmondsworth: Penguin

2. See: Baker, E., and Newnes, C. (2005). The discourse of responsibility. In. C. Newnes and N. Radcliffe (eds.) *Making and Breaking Children's Lives.* Ross-on-Wye: PCCS Books 30-39

3. Szasz, T. (1994). *Cruel Compassion: Psychiatric control of society's unwanted.* New York: John Wiley & Sons p.156

4. Vasan, N., Chaudhary, N.P., Aragam, G.G., Nagpal, A., Mckenzie, T., and Chen, C. (2017). Technological Ventures Offer New Hope for the Future of Psychiatry. http://www.psychiatrictimes.com/special-reports/technological-ventures-offer-new-hope-future-psychiatry?GUID=E7BD9D7E-A63B-41ED-A97F-34FCBFAAE3D6&rememberme=1&ts=04012018 December 25, 2017 | Special Reports, Telepsychiatry Retrieved; 5th January, 2018

5. See: Fitzpatrick K, Darcy A, Vierhile M.(2017). Delivering cognitive behaviour therapy to young adults

with symptoms of depression and anxiety using a fully automated conversational agent (Woebot): a randomized controlled trial. *JMIR Ment Health*. 4:e19. and Romeo N. (2016).The chatbot will see you now. *The New Yorker*. December 25, 2016. https://www.newyorker.com/tech/elements/the-chatbot-will-see-you-now. Accessed November 6, 2017.

6. https://www.blog.google/products/search/learning-more-about-clinical-depression-phq-9-questionnaire Retrieved; 4th January, 2018

7. See, *Psychiatric Times* psychiatrictimes@email.cmpmedica-usa.com

8. Rosario, V. A. (1997) *The Erotic Imagination: French histories of perversity*. New York: Oxford University Press

9. https://en.wikipedia/ St. Patrick's Hospital Retrieved 12th February 2018

10. O'Donoghue, E.G. (1915). *The Story of Bethlehem Hospital, from its Foundation in 1247*. New York: Dutton. p.250

11. Swift, J. (1704) *A Tale of a Tub*. In. A. Ross and D. Woolley (eds.) (1984). *Jonathan Swift* pp. 62-164, 147-148 for quote. Oxford: Oxford University Press.

12. Gaskell, E. (1848). *Mary Barton. Tale of Manchester Life*. London: Chapman & Hall

13. Chekhov, A. (1892) Ward No.6. In. Chekhov, A. (1963) *Seven Short Stories by Chekhov*. trans by B. Makanowitzky. New York: Bantam Books.

14. Szasz op.cit. see, Note 3 p.116

15. Barker, P. (1991) *Regeneration*. New York: Viking Press (Penguin edition)

16. *Seksik, Laurent (2013). Le cas Eduard Einstein* (French ed.). Paris: Flammarion. pp. 128–131

17. Carr, C. (1994). *The Alienist*. London: Little, Brown and Company

18. Lessing to Roberta Rubenstein, 28 March 1977, quoted in Rubenstein, R. (1979) *The Novelistic Vision of Doris Lessing* Urbana: University of Illinois Press p. 197. Quoted in. Showalter, E. (1987) *The Female Malady: Women, madness and English culture, 1830-1980*. London: Virago p. 238

19. Showalter, E. (1987) *The Female Malady: Women, madness and English culture, 1830-1980*. London: Virago p. 238-241

Opposition and Oprah Winfrey

1. Formerly The Prevention of Professional Abuse Network (POPAN) Witness campaigns for professional bodies to develop standardised complaints procedures which are sensitive to the possible distress caused to patients . Witness runs a helpline for patients who have been abused: a third of callers claim to have been abused by counsellors or psychotherapists. http://www.wherecanifind.net/cgi-bin/callentry.cgi?255 (retrieved 15 March 2015).

2. See: http://intcamp.wordpress.com/ban-ect/ and http://camhjournal. com/2012/04/24/2004-a-campaign-against-direct-ect/

3. See, for example, ECT Global Support https://www.facebook.com/groups/414257 808688052/ and Mind Freedom Ireland http://www.mindfreedomireland.com/

4. Szasz, T (1987). *Insanity: The idea and its consequences.* New York: Wiley

5. Unzicker, R. (1989). My own. A personal journey through madness and re-emergence. *Psychosocial Rehabilitation Journal, 13,* 71-75 p.71

6. https://www.youtube.com/watch?v=F4WygjHKA8k

7. Chamberlain, J. (1977). *On Our Own: Patient controlled alternatives to the mental health system.* New York: Hawthorn

8. Lindow, V. (1999) Survivor-controlled alternatives to psychiatric services. In. C. Newnes, G. Holmes and C. Dunn. (eds.) *This is Madness: A critical look at psychiatry and the future of mental health services.* Monmouth: PCCS Books

9. http://www.enusp.org/.

10. Hölling, I. (1998) Ämterwahn. In. K. Kempker (ed.). *Flucht in die Wirklichkeit.* Berlin: Peter Lehmann Antipsychiatrieverlag, pp.149–158; Hölling, I. (1999) Three years of anti-psychiatric practice at the Berlin Runaway-House. *Changes: An International Journal of Psychology and Psychotherapy, 17, 4,* 278–288 and Wehde, U. (1992). The Runaway-House: Human support instead of inhuman psychiatric treatment. *Changes: An International Journal of Psychology and Psychotherapy, 10, 2,* 154–160.

11. http://www.mentalhealthy.co.uk/news/379-oprah-shocked-that-electroconvulsive-therapy-ect-still-used-today.html Retrieved January 17th 2018

12. Depression Treatment Breakthroughs, Beyond ECT-Oprah.com

Precision and Mervyn Peake

1. Weiner, D.B. (1994) Le geste de Pinel: the history of a psychiatric myth. In. M.Micale and R.Porter (eds) *Discovering the History of Psychiatry*. Oxford: OUP pp 232-247

2. Digby, A. (1985). *Madness, Morality and Medicine: A study of the York Retreat, 1796–1914*. Cambridge: Cambridge University Press, pp. 78–82.

3. Allderidge, P. (1985). Bedlam: fact or fantasy? In. W.F. Bynum, Roy Porter, and M. Shepherd (eds) *The Anatomy of Madness: Vol II Institutions and Society*. London: Tavistock

4. Fennel, P. (1996). *Treatment Without Consent: Law, psychiatry and the treatment of mentally disordered people since 1845*. London: Routledge p.14 Fennel adds in a footnote (p.302) that Allderidge found Norris's extreme form of restraint to be a response to his violence and dangerousness since his admission in 1800. He was first restrained in the cage in 1804 and remained in it for nine years.

5. *Ibid*. p. 14

6. Valenstein, E. (1986). *Great and Desperate Cures: The rise and decline of psychosurgery and other radical treatments for mental illness*. New York: Basic Books and Shorter, E. (1997) *A History of Psychiatry: From the era of the asylum to the age of Prozac*. Chichester: John Wiley & Sons

7. Shorter, E. and Healy, D. (2007) *Shock Therapy: A History of Electroconvulsive Treatment in Mental Illness*. New Brunswick, NJ: Rutgers University Press . p.41

[8] *Ibid.* p.181

[9] Sadowsky, J. (2017). *Electroconvulsive Therapy in America: The Anatomy of a Medical Controversy.* London: Routledge

[10] Hirshbein, L. (2012). Electroconvulsive therapy, memory, and self in America. *J Hist Neuroscience. 21,* 147-169.

[11] http://www.psychiatrictimes.com/ history-psychiatry/ect-history-psychiatric-controversy/page/0/2 Retrieved 25 January, 2018.

[12] Carpenter, L.L., Janicak, P.G., Aaronson, S.T., Boyadjis, T., Brock, D.G., Cook, I.A., Dunner, D.L., Lanocha, K., Solvason, H.B., and Demitrack, M.A. (2012). Transcranial magnetic stimulation (TMS) for major depression: a multisite, naturalistic, observational study of acute treatment outcomes in clinical practice. *Depression and Anxiety. 29(7):*587-96. doi: 10.1002/da.21969. Epub 2012 Jun 11. https://www.ncbi.nlm.nih.gov/pubmed/22689344 Retrieved. 26th December, 2016

[13] Davis, N. (2015). A new milestone in non-pharmaceutical treatments for depression https://www.theguardian.com/science/head-quarters/2015/may/18/non-pharmaceutical-treatments-for-depression-magstim-tms Retrieved. 5th February 2018

[14] Hervey, N. (1985). A slavish bowing down: the Lunacy Commission and the psychiatric profession. In. W.F. Bynum, R. Porter and M. Shepherd (eds.) *The Anatomy of Madness Vol. II: Institutions and society.* London: Tavistock Publications pp.98-131 p.104

321

15. Rosario, V. A. (1997).*The Erotic Imagination: French histories of perversity.* New York: Oxford University Press

16. Stein, D. B. (2012). *The Psychology Industry under a Microscope!* Plymouth, UK: University Press of America Inc., p. 33

17. Kelley, J.L. (1996). *Psychiatric Malpractice. Stories of Patients, Psychiatrists and the Law.* New Brunswick, NJ: Rutgers University Press. p.207

18. Demetrios S. J. (2003). Dementia With Lewy Bodies and the Neurobehavioral Decline of Mervyn Peake *Arch Neurol.* 60(6):889-892

19. Peake, M. (1972/1974). The Threads Remain. From: *A Book of Nonsense.* (Originally published 1972) London: Pan Books. p.82

Queerness

1.Broude, G. and Greene, S.J. (1976). Cross-cultural codes on twenty sexual attitudes and practices. *Ethnology, 15,* (4), 409-429

2. Mártir de Anleriá, P. (1530). *Décadas del Mundo Nuevo.* Quoted by Coello de la Rosa, A. (2002). 'Good Indians', 'Bad Indians', 'What Christians?': The Dark Side of the New World in Gonzalo Fernández de Oviedo y Valdés (1478–1557), *Delaware Review of Latin American Studies*, Vol. 3, No. 2

3. Foucault, M. (1986). Of Other Spaces. trans. J. Miskowiec, *Diacritics Spring*: 22-27

4. Tulchin, A.A. (2007). Same-Sex Couples Creating Households in Old Regime France: The Uses of the Affrèrement, *The Journal of Modern History. 79,* (3)

613 647

5. Gladfelder, H. (2006). *In Search of Lost Texts: Thomas Cannon's 'Ancient and Modern Pederasty Investigated and Exemplified'* University of London: Institute of Historical Research

6. See, Grosskurth, P. (1980). *Havelock Ellis: A biography.* London: Allen Lane

7. Fathi, N. (2007). Despite Denials, Gays Insist They Exist, if Quietly, in Iran. *New York Times. September 30* Retrieved 1st October 2007

8. Grosskurth op. cit. p.188

9. Grosskurth op. cit. p.231

10. Ellis, H. & Symonds, J.A. (1897). *Sexual Inversion: Studies in the psychology of sex.* Wilson and Macmillan: Harvard.

11. von Kraft-Ebbing, R. (1892). *Psychopathia Sexualis* (trans. C.G. Chaddock, from 7th German edition). Philadelphia: F.A. Davis.

12. Wolpe, J. (1973). *The Practice of Behavior Therapy* 2nd ed. Oxford, England: Pergamon.

13. American Psychiatric Association. (1952). *Diagnostic and statistical manual of mental disorders* (1st ed.). APA

14. American Psychiatric Association. (1968). *Diagnostic and statistical manual of mental disorders* (2nd ed.). APA

15. Berke, J.H. (2015). *The Hidden Freud: His Hassidic roots.* London: Karnac Book

16. Freud, S. (1905/1962).*Three Essays on the Theory of Sexuality.* Drei Abhandlungen zur Sexualtheorie. Trans. J. Strachey New York: Basic Books

17. Freud, S. (1926/1959). *The Question of Lay Analysis.* Trans. J. Strachey in the Standard Edition. London: Hogarth Press and the Institute of Psycho-Analysis

18. Smith, G., Bartlett, A., & King, M. (2004). Treatments of homosexuality in Britain since the 1950s - an oral history: the experience of patients. *British Medical Journal, 328*, 427-429

19. Haldeman, D.C. (1991). Sexual Orientation Conversion Therapy for Gay Men and Lesbians: A Scientific Examination in Homosexuality. In J.C. Gonsiorek, & J.D. Weinrich (eds.) *Research Implications for Public Practice.* Newbury Park, C.A.: Sage. http://doi.org/10.4135/9781483325422

20. Smith et al. op. cit.

21. Dickenson, T. (2014). *'Curing Queers': Mental Nurses and their patients 1935-74.* Manchester University Press: Manchester.

22. Schwartz, S. (1998). The role of values in the nature/nurture debate about psychiatric disorders. *Social Psychiatry and Epidemiological Psychiatry, 33,* 356–362.

23. American Psychiatric Association. (1973). *Diagnostic and statistical manual of mental disorders* (2nd ed. 7th Revision). APA

Research and Robeson

1. Turner, K. (2018). *Psychotherapy: A critical examination.* Monmouth: PCCS Books

2. Stein, D. B. (2012). *The Psychology Industry under a Microscope!* Plymouth, UK: University Press of America Inc., p. 1.

3. Sandison, R. (2001). *A Century of Psychiatry, Psychotherapy and Group Analysis: A search for integration*. London: Jessica Kingsley Publishers p. 49

4. Martin, J. (1962). The treatment of 12 male homosexuals with LSD. *Acta Psychotherapeutica, 10*, 394-402

5. See: Boyle, D. (2016). *Ronald Laing: The rise and fall and rise of a revolutionary psychiatrist*. London: The Real Press

6. Sandison, R. (2001). op.cit. p. 53

7. Eranti, S. & McLoughlin, D. M. (2003). Electroconvulsive therapy – state of the art. *British Journal of Psychiatry, 182*, 8–9.

7. Brus, O., Pia Nordanskog, P., Båve, U., Cao, Y., Hammar, Å., Landén, M. Lundberg, J., and Axel Nordenskjöld, A. (2017). Subjective Memory Immediately Following Electroconvulsive Therapy *The Journal of ECT, 33*(2):96–103,

8. Ziegelmayer, C., Hajak, G., Bauer, A., Held, M., Rupprecht;, R., and Trapp,W. (2017). Cognitive Performance Under Electroconvulsive Therapy (ECT) in ECT-Naive Treatment-Resistant Patients With Major Depressive Disorder *The Journal of ECT,* 33(2):104–110

9. Kerner, N. and Prudic, J. (2014). Current electroconvulsive therapy practice and research in the geriatric population. *Neuropsychiatry, 4*, (1), 33–54.

10. Greenhalgh, J., Knight, C., Hind, D., Beverley, C. & Walters, S. (2005). Clinical and cost-effectiveness of electroconvulsive therapy for depressive illness, schizophrenia, catatonia and mania: Systematic reviews

and economic modelling studies. *Health Technology Assessment, Mar, 9 (9),* 1–156, iii–iv, p. 9.

[11.] Ross, C.A. (2006). The Sham ECT Literature: Implications for consent to ECT. *Ethical Human Psychology and Psychiatry, 8, 1,* 17-28 p.26

[12.] Buchan,H., Johnstone,E., McPherson,K., Palmer,R.L., Crow,T.J., & Brandon,S. (1992). Who benefits from electroconvulsive therapy? *British Journal of Psychiatry, 160,* 355–359. p.359 In. Johnstone, L. (2003). A shocking treatment? *The Psychologist, 16,5,* 236-239

[13.] See: Green, N.E. and Swiontkowski, M.F. (2009). *Skeletal Trauma in Children Vol 3*. 4th Ed. Philadelphia: Saunders/Elsevier

[14.] Brown, E. N, Lydic, R. and Schiff, N. D. (2010). General anesthesia, sleep, and coma. *New England Journal of Medicine, Vol. 363,* December, pp. 2638-50.

[15.] Kellner, C. and Iosifescu, D.V. (2017). Ketamine and ECT: better alone than together? *Lancet Psychiatry, 4,* (5), 348-349 http://www.thelancet.com/journals/lanpsy/article/PII S2215-0366(17)30099-8/fulltext Accessed 27th February 2018

[16.] Anderson, I. M., Blamire, A., Branton, T., Clark, R., Downey, D., Dunn, G.,Easton, A., Elliott, R., Elwell, C., Hayden, K., Holland, F., Karim, S., Loo, C., Lowe, J., Nair, R., Oakley, T., Prakash, P.K., Williams, S.R., and McAllister-Williams,R.H. (on behalf of the 8 member Ketamine-ECT Study Team) (2016). Ketamine augmentation of electroconvulsive therapy to improve neuropsychological and clinical outcomes in depression

(Ketamine-ECT): a multicentre, double-blind, randomised, parallel-group, superiority trial. *European Neuropsychopharmacology,* *26,* Suppl. 2. The 'Ketamine-ECT study Service User Group (Study team)' was made up of six service survivors from the north-west of England. It aimed to provide input into patient information materials, the recruitment process, and exclusion criteria and participated in Research Assistant training.

[17.] Comparing Electroconvulsive Therapy and Ketamine Treatment for Adults with Major Depression That Has Not Responded to Antidepressant Medicines https://www.pcori.org/research-results/2016/comparing-electroconvulsive-therapy-and-ketamine-treatment-adults-major Accessed 28 February 2018.

[18.] Johnstone, L. (2003). ECT: A shocking treatment? *The Psychologist May Vol 16 No 5* 236-9

[19,] See, for example: McLoughlin, D. M., Mogg, A., Eranti, S., Pluck, G., Purvis, R., Edwards, D., Landau, S., Brown, R., Rabe-Heskith, S., Howard, R., Philpot, M., Rothwell, J., Romeo, R., and Knapp, M. (2007). The clinical effectiveness and cost of repetitive transcranial magnetic stimulation versus electroconvulsive therapy in severe depression: a multicentre pragmatic randomised controlled trial and economic analysis. *Health Technology Assessment 11(24)* 1-54.

[20.]https://www.google.co.uk/search?q=cost+of+ect+uk&oq=cost+of+ECT+&aqs=chrome.1.69i57j0l5.12048j0j8&sourceid=chrome&ie=UTF-8

[21] Greenhalgh et al., op.cit.

[22] Vallejo-Torres,L., Castilla, I., González, N., Hunter, R., Serrano-Pérez, P., and Perestelo-Pérez, L. (2015). Cost-effectiveness of electroconvulsive therapy compared to repetitive transcranial magnetic stimulation for treatment-resistant severe depression: a decision model. *Psychological Medicine, 45,* (7), 1459–1470. Published online 2014 Oct 30. doi: 10.1017/S0033291714002554

[23] Duckworth, K. (2009). National Alliance on Mental Illness: American Indian and Alaska Native women and depression FACT SHEET: What are the risk factors for American Indian and Alaskan Native women? Available at http://www2.nami.org/ Template.cfm?Section=Women_and_Depression&Template=/ContentManagement/ ContentDisplay.cfm&ContentID=88885 Retrieved 16th March, 2015

[24] See, for example, Dillard, D. A., Smith, J. J., Ferucci, E. D. & Lanier, A. P. (2012). Depression prevalence and associated factors among Alaska native people: The Alaska Education and Research Towards Health (Earth) study. *Journal of Affective Disorders, 136,* (3) 1088–1097.

[25] Enns, M.W. and Reiss, J.P. (2015). *Canadian Psychiatric Association Position Paper* March 16, 2015 https://ww1.cpa-apc.org/Publications/Position_Papers/Therapy.asp Retrieved 28th February, 2018

[26] https://www.fisherwallace.com/pages/safety-and-efficacy-of-cranial-electrotherapy-stimulation

Retrieved 28th February, 2018

27. The 'gift relationship' between patients and physician makes the expression of gratitude for a prescribed drug or a prescription of electroshock more probable than any complaint. In simple terms the patient shares intimate information with the prescriber who, in a socially normative way, returns the favour via the 'gift' of inscription and prescription. Any admission that the drug has not been taken due to adverse effects or the electroshock has failed may not come until after many similar consultations.

28. See, for example, Szasz, T.S. (1981). *Sex: Facts, Fraud and Follies*. Oxford: Basil Blackwell

29. Moncrieff, J., Rapley, M. & Timimi, S. (2011). The construction of psychiatric diagnoses: The case of adult ADHD. *Journal of Critical Psychology, Counselling and Psychotherapy*, *11, 1*, 16-28. Quoted in. Rapley, M. (2018). Sigmund and Michel, Alain and Mary Go Shopping: The commodification of misery. *Journal of Critical Psychology, Counselling and Psychotherapy, 18, 1,* 30-38

30. Bhanji, N.H.,, Baron, D.A., Benjamin, D.A., Lacy, W., Gross, L. S., Goin, M.K., Sumner, C.R., Fischer, B.A. & Slaby, A.E. (2008). Direct-to-Consumer Marketing: An Attitude survey of psychiatric physicians. *Primary Psychiatry,15,11*:67-71.

31. Kaiser Family Foundation (2003). *Impact of Direct-to-Consumer Advertising on Prescription Drug Spending*. Henry J. Kaiser Family Foundation: Menlo Park, CA. Available from: ww.kff.org/rxdrugs/upload/Impact-of-Direct-to-

Consumer-Advertising-on-Prescription-Drug-
Spending-Summary-of-Findings.pdf (p. 5)

32. See: Newnes, C. (2016). The Oblivion Express: Big Pharma. In. C. Newnes. *Inscription, Diagnosis and Deception in the Mental Health Industry: How Psy governs us all.* Basingstoke: Palgrave Macmillan pp.81-106

33. https://www.uptodate.com/contents/electroconvulsi ve-therapy-ect-beyond-the-basics   Retrieved,   27th February, 2018

34. https://ectstatistics.wordpress.com/2013/01/13/paul -robesons-ect-at-the-priory/ Retrieved, 27th January, 2018

Sadism and Spike Milligan

1. See; Newnes, C. (2014). *Clinical Psychology: A critical examination.* Ross on Wye: PCCS p.142

2. Abse, D.W. and Ewing, J.A. (1956). Transference and countertransference in somatic therapies. *J Nerv Mental Disease, 123*(1):32-40.

3. http://www.carolinephillips.net/articles/archive/new spapers/evening-standard/murder-madness-and-milligan.html Retrieved; January 12th 2018

4. *Ibid.*

Torture

1. http://www.dailykos.com/story/2014/12/09/1350553 /-CIA-paid-two-ex-mili tary-psychologists-who-helped-designed-and-run-torture-program-81-million# Retrieved 25 February 2015.

2. http://www.intelligence.senate.gov/study2014/sscistu

dy1.pdf. Retrieved 25th February 2015.

3. It is worth noting that the brain biochemical imbalance theory of depression has been quietly dropped in public statements from the Royal College of Psychiatrists over the last ten years or so. Despite that, the notion has so taken root that people taking psycho-active drugs frequently refer to the imbalance. See, Unhappiness and the Unknown.

4. Scull, A. (1990). Desperate remedies: A Gothic tale of madness and modern medicine. In. R.M. Murray and T.H. Turner (eds.) *Lectures on the History of Psychiatry: The Squibb Series.* London: Gaskell/Royal College of Psychiatrists pp.144-169

5. *Ibid.* p.153

6. *Ibid.* p.154

7. Lewis, B.G. (1922). The winning fight against mental disease. *Review of Reviews,* December. In. Scull op. cit. p. 156

8. Scull op. cit. p.166

9. Cromby, J. (2004) Depression: Embodying social inequality. *Journal of Critical Psychology, Counselling and Psychotherapy, 4, 3*, 176–186, p.177.

10. Cromby, J. (2006). Reconstructing the person. *Clinical Psychology Forum, 162,* 13–16.

11. Hale. E., (2009). Child shock therapy. January 25, http://intcamp.wordpress .com/ect-kids/. Retrieved 8 September 2014 (International Campaign to Ban Electroshock). Link: http://www.news.com.au/heraldsun/story/0, 21985,24958938-2862,00.html.

12. Mental Disability Rights International (2005) Behind

Closed Doors: Human Rights Abuses in the Psychiatric Facilities, Orphanages and Rehabilitation Centers of Turkey. MDRI. www.youtube.com/watch?v=Q9lNUsLLC8c

13. Lynch, T. (2004). *Beyond Prozac: Healing mental distress*. Llangarron: PCCS Books

14. Fanon, F. (1965). *A Dying Colonialism* NY: Grove Press. p.138

15. http://www.freedommag.org/issue/201411-held-back/reform/shock-treatment-truth-behind-electroshock-therapy.html Retrieved 14th February, 2018

16. *We're Not Mad, We're Angry*. Channel 4 'Eleventh Hour' documentary made in 1986. Available at www.youtube. com/watch?v=qD36m1mveoY Retrieved 17th March 2015).

Unhappiness and the Unknown

1. Stimmel, B. (1983). *Pain, Analgesia and Addiction*. New York: Raven Press. Cited in: Gabe, J. (ed.) (1991) *Understanding Tranquilliser Use: The Role of the Social Sciences*. London: Routledge, p.2.

2. Gabe, J. (ed.) (1991). *Understanding Tranquilliser Use: The Role of the Social Sciences*. London: Routledge, pp.2-4

3. Retrieved 1 June 2013 from http://www.ect.org/famous-shock-patients/

5. Marsella, A.J. (1980). Depressive experience and disorder across cultures. In. Harry C. Triandis et al. (eds.) *Handbook of Cross-cultural Psychology*, 6 vols. Boston: Allyn and Bacon 6: 237-289, pages 274 and 261

respectively. Quoted in: Jackson, S.W. (1986). *Melancholia and Depression: From Hippocrates to Modern Times.* New Haven and London: Yale University Press. p.244

6. Raleigh, W. (1909/2015). *William Shakespeare.* London: Leopold Classic Library

7. Boyle, D. (2000). *The Tyranny of Numbers: Why counting can't make us happy.* London: Harper Collins

8. Newnes, C. (2001). Speaking out. *Ethical Human Sciences and Services, 3, 1,* 135-142

9. Woods, J. (2018). Depressed patients don't need pills – just the right ones. *The Daily Telegraph,* 23rd February p.21

Vested interest and Vaslav Nijinsky

1. Editorial (1997). What is psychiatry? *American Journal of Psychiatry, 154* (5) 591–593, p. 593.

2. Zappa, F. (1982). 'Single Release' – liner notes for *Ship Arriving Too Late to Save a Drowning Witch.* Los Angeles: Barking Pumpkin Records

3. W.H.O. (2015). http://www.who.int/trade/glossary/story073/en/. Retrieved 20th February 2015.

4. http://projects.propublica.org/docdollars/. Retrieved 20th February 2015

5. Grohol, J.M. (2011). Top 50 Psychiatrists Paid by Pharmaceutical Companies. http://psychcentral.com/blog/archives/2010/10/23/top-50-psychiatrists-paid -by-pharmaceutical-companies/. Retrieved 20th February 2015. See also; Wood, S. and Lowes, R. (2010). Psychiatrists Dominate

'Doctor-Dollars' Database Listing Big Pharma Payments. http://www.medscape.com/viewarticle/731028. Retrieved 23rd February 2015.

6. Breggin, P. (1991). *Toxic Psychiatry: Why therapy, empathy and love must replace the drugs, electroshock and biochemical theories of the 'new psychiatry.'* New York: St. Martin's Press. Quoted in Johnstone, L. (1994). Values in human services. *Care in Place: The International Journal of Networks and Community, 1, 1,* 3-8 p. 7

7. Lay, K. (2018). NHS fails to declare drug firm cash. *The Times*, January 4th 2018

8. Shorter, E. and Healy, D. (2007). *Shock Therapy: A history of electroconvulsive treatment in mental illness.* New Brunswick, NJ: Rutgers University Press

9. Cameron, D. G. (1994). Sham statistics, the myth of convulsive therapy and the case for consumer misinformation. *The Journal of Mind and Behavior, 15, 1 and 2,* 177-198 pp.180-1

Women

1. https://en.wikipedia.org/wiki/Sati_(practice)#Modern_times Retrieved 20th February 2018

2. National Inquiry into the Separation of Aboriginal and Torres Strait Islander Children from Their Families (1997). *Bringing Them Home: Report of the national inquiry into the separation of Aboriginal and Torres Strait Islander children from their families.* Sydney: Human Rights and Equal Opportunity Commission, Commonwealth of Australia p.37 Cited in: Dudgeon, P.,

Cubillo, C., and Bray, A. (2015). The stolen generations: The forced removal of First Peoples' children in Australia In C. Newnes (ed.) *Children in Society: Politics, policies and interventions* Monmouth: PCCS Books pp.50-81

3. Fickling, D. (2005). 'One in three blames women for being raped', *The Guardian*, Monday November 21st

4. Though consistent with Nyirö's original speculations (see; History and Hemingway) concerning an antagonistic relationship between schizophrenia and epilepsy, the use of electroshock with those inscribed with schizophrenia is no more justified by the evidence base than it is with people called depressed.

5. Faith, K. (1993). *Unruly Women: The politics of confinement & resistance.* Vancouver: Press Gang Publishers

6. Gartrell, N., Herman, J., Olarte, S., Feldstein, M. and Localio. R. (1986). Psychiatrist-patient sexual contact: Results of a national survey. *American Journal of Psychiatry, 143,* 1126–1131. Gartrell, N., Herman, J., Olarte, S., Feldstein, M. and Localio, R. (1987). Psychiatrist-patient sexual contact: Results of a national survey. *American Journal of Psychiatry, 144,* 164–169.

7. Sackeim, H.A., Prudic, J., Fuller, R., Keilp, J., Lavori, P.W. and Olfson, M. (2007). The cognitive effects of electroconvulsive therapy in community settings. *Neuropsychopharmacology, 32, 1,* 244–154.

8. Burstow, B. (2006). Electroshock as a form of violence against women. *Violence Against Women, 12, 4,* 372–392

9. Hale. E., (2009) Child shock therapy. January 25, http://intcamp.wordpress .com/ect-kids/. (International Campaign to Ban Electroshock). Link: http://www.news.com.au/heraldsun/story/0, 21985,24958938-2862,00.html. Retrieved 8th September 2014

10. http://www.ect.org/resources/california.html Retrieved 30th May, 2013

11. Reid, W. H., Keller, S., Leatherman, M. & Mason, M. (1998). ECT in Texas: 19 months of mandatory reporting. *Journal of Clinical Psychiatry, 59* (1), 8–13, p. 13.

12. http://ectstatistics.wordpress.com/2013/01/30/ectwithout-consent-in-england-201112/ Retrieved 30th May, 2013

13. SEAN, (2011). *Scottish ECT Accreditation Network Annual Report 2011. A summary of ECT in Scotland for 2010.* Edinburgh: Scottish ECT Accreditation Network.

14. Davis, N. (2017). Electroconvulsive therapy mostly used on women and older people, says study. *The Guardian* 20 Oct.

15. Newnes, C. (2001). Speaking out. *Ethical Human Sciences and Services, 3, 1,* 135-142

16. Fennell, P. (1996). *Treatment Without Consent: Law, psychiatry and the treatment of mentally disordered people since 1845.* London: Routledge pp. 66-72

17. Despite his liberal (though decidedly paternalistic) views on sexuality Havelock Ellis termed masturbation 'Auto-Erotism' and suggested it led to nervous

disorders. In the second edition of *Handbuch der Sexualwissenschaften* by Moll he was recommending a masturbatory prophylactic - Onaniebandagen; suits of armour fitted over the male or female genitals and attached to a locked belt- first proposed by Lajade-Lafond in 1830. See; Marcus, S. (1966). *The Other Victorians*. London: Weidenfeld & Nicolson

[18.]https://www.medicalnewstoday.com/articles/317768.php Retrieved 3rd March 2018

[19.] Cooper, D. (1978). *The Language of Madness*. London: Allen Lane p.74.

[20.] Morris, R. T. (1892). Is evolution trying to do away with the clitoris? *Transaction of the American Association of Obstetricians and Gynecologists, 5,* 288-302. Cited in Johnsdottre, S. (2012).Projected Cultural Histories of the Cutting of Female Genitalia: A Poor Reflection as in a Mirror *History and Anthropology, 23*, 1, 91-114

X-rays

[1.] Christmas, D., & Matthews, K. (2016). Neurosurgical Treatments for Patients with Chronic, Treatment-Refractory Depression: A Retrospective, Consecutive, Case Series Comparison of Anterior Capsulotomy, Anterior. Cingulotomy and Vagus Nerve Stimulation. *Stereotactic and Functional Neurosurgery, 93* (6), 387-392

[2.] Scull, A. (1990). Desperate remedies: A Gothic tale of madness and modern medicine. In. R.M. Murray and T.H. Turner (eds.) *Lectures on the History of Psychiatry: The Squibb Series.* London: Gaskell/Royal

College of Psychiatrists pp.144-169 p. 152

3. Luxenburg, J.S., Swedo, S.E., Flament, M.E., Friedland, R.P., Rapaport, J., and Rapaport, S. (1988). Neuroanatomical abnormalities in obsessive compulsive disorder detected with quantative x-ray computed tomography. *American Journal of Psychiatry 145,* 1089-1093

4. Baughman, F. (2006). *The ADHD Fraud: How psychiatry makes patients of normal children.* Oxford: Trafford Press.

5. Omran, A.R., Shore, R.E., Markoff, R. A., Friedhoff, A., Albert, R.E., Barr, H, Dahlstrom, W.G., and Pasternack, B.S. (1978). Follow-up study of patients treated by X-ray epilation for tinea capitis: psychiatric and psychometric evaluation. *Am J Public Health. 68* (6): 561–567.

6. Neuman, F. (2018) Fighting Fear: *A Misunderstanding Central to OCD* https://www.psychologytoday.com/blog/fighting-fear/201603/misunderstanding-central-ocd Retrieved 23rd February 2018

7. Chanpattana, W. and Kramer, B.A. (2004). Electroconvulsive therapy practice in Thailand. *Journal of Electroconvulsive Therapy, 20,* (2), 94-98

8. Kalinowsky, L.B. (1967). The convulsive therapies. In. A.M. Freedman and H.I. Kaplan (eds.) *Comprehensive Textbook of Psychiatry.* Baltimore: Wilkins & Wilkins. pp. 1279-1285

Youngsters

1. Boyle, D. (2000). *The Tyranny of Numbers: Why*

counting can't make us happy. London: Harper Collins.

2. Werry, J.S. (1992). Child psychiatric disorders: Are they classifiable? *British Journal of Psychiatry, 161,* 472-480 p.478

3. Taylor, J.H. (1990). Tranquillizers anyone? *Forbes,* December 10th 214-216 p.216

4. Szasz, T. (1994). *Cruel Compassion: Psychiatric control of society's unwanted.* New York: John Wiley & Sons p.83

5. *Ibid.*

6. Newnes, C. (2015). Chapter three. In *Inscription, Diagnosis and Deception in the Mental Health Industry: How Psy governs us all.* Basingstoke: Palgrave Macmillan.

7. Bender, L. (1947). One hundred cases of childhood schizophrenia treated with electric shock. *Transactions of the American Neurological Society, 72,* 165–169. Quoted in Rey, J. M. & Walter, G. (1997). Half a century of ECT use in young people. *The American Journal of Psychiatry, 154,* (5) 595–602, p. 596.

8. Shorter, E. & Healy, D. (2007). *Shock Therapy: A history of electroconvulsive treatment in mental illness.* New Brunswick, NJ: Rutgers University Press, p. 137.

9. Boodman, S. G. (1996). Shock therapy: It's back. *Washington Post,* 24 September, 14–20.

10. Decker, H. (2013). The Making of DSM-IIIRG: A Diagnostic Manual's conquest of American psychiatry, Oxford: Oxford University Press.

11. Wikipedia (n.d.). Lauretta Bender. Available at

http://www.en.wikipedia.org/wiki/ Lauretta_Bender (retrieved 9 March 2015).

12. Rey, J. M. & Walter, G. (1997). Half a century of ECT use in young people. *American Journal of Psychiatry, 154* (5) 595–602.

13. Cohen, D., Paillère-Martinot, M. L., & Basquin, M. (1997). Use of electroconvulsive therapy in adolescents. *Convulsive Therapy, 13* (1) 25–31.

14. Arscott, K. (1999). ECT: The facts psychiatry declines to mention. In C. Newnes, G. Holmes and C. Dunn (eds.) *This is Madness: A critical look at psychiatry and the future of mental health services.* pp. 97–118 Ross-on-Wye: PCCS Books.

15. Wachtel, L. E., Dhossche, D. M. & Kellner, C. H. (2011). When is electroconvulsive therapy appropriate for children and adolescents? *Medical Hypotheses, 76* (3) 395–399.

16. Zaw, F.K.M., Bates, G.D.L., Murali, V., et al. (1999). Catatonia, autism and ECT. *Developmental Medicine and Child Neurology, 41,* 843–845. Quoted in Muir, P. J. (2005). *The use of ECT in people with learning disability.* In A.I.F. Scott (ed.) *The ECT Handbook, Second Edition: The third report of the Royal College of Psychiatrists' Special Committee on ECT* (pp. 57–67). Gaskell: RCP p. 62.

17. Bloch, Y., Levcovitch, Y., Bloch, A. M. & Mendlovic, S. (2001). Electroconvulsive therapy in adolescents: Similarities to and differences from adults. *Journal of the American Academy of Child and Adolescent Psychiatry, 40* (11) 1332–1336.

18. Willoughby, C. L., Hradek, E. A. & Richards, N. R.

(1997). Use of electroconvulsive therapy with children: An overview and case report. *Journal of Child and Adolescent Psychiatric Nursing, 10* (3) 11–17.

[19.] Calev, A. (1994). Neuropsychology and ECT: Past and future research trends. *Psychopharmacological Bulletin, 30*, 461–469.

[20.] Parmar, R (1993). Attitudes of child psychiatrists to electroconvulsive therapy. *Psychiatric Bulletin, 17,* 12–13.

[21.] Paillère-Martinot, M. L., Zivi, A. & Basquin, M. (1990). Utilisation de l'ECT chez l'adolescent. *Encéphale, 16* (5) 399–404.

[22.] Hale. E., (2009) Child shock therapy. January 25, http://intcamp.wordpress .com/ect-kids/. Retrieved 8 September 2014 (International Campaign to Ban Electroshock).http://www.news.com.au/heraldsun/story/0, 21985,24958938-2862,00.html.

[23.] Conselho Federal de Medicina (Brazilian Federal Council of Medicine) (2002). Resolução CFM Nº 1640/2002. Dispõe sobre a eletroconvulsoterapia e dá outras providências [PubMed Abstract]. Brasília: CFM.

[24.] Lima, N.N.R., Nascimento, V. B., Peixoto, J.A.C., Moreira, M. M., Neto, M.L.R., Almeida, J. C., Vasconcelos, C.A.C., Teixeira, S. A., Júnior, J. G., Junior, F.T.C., Guimarães, D.D.M., Brasil, A. Q., Cartaxo, J. S., Akerman, M. & Reis, A.O.A. (2013). Electroconvulsive therapy use in adolescents: A systematic review. *Annals of General Psychiatry 12* (17). Available at http://www.annals-general-psychiatry.com/content/12/1/17 (retrieved 1 May 2015). Lima et al use the PRISMA protocol for their analysis. See Moher, D., Liberati, A., Tetzlaff, I. & Altman, D. G. (2009). Preferred reporting items for systematic reviews and meta-analyses: The PRISMA statement. PLoS Med, 6, (7) e10097.

[25.] *Ibid.*

[26.] AACAP Official Action (2004). Practice Parameter for Use of Electroconvulsive Therapy with Adolescents. *Journal of the American Academy of Child and Adolescent Psychiatry, 43,* (12) 1521–1539. The authors claim that 'mood disorders' have a high rate of response to electroshock (75–100%); 'psychotic disorders' have a lower response rate (50–60%). See also; Salleh M. A., Papakostas, I., Zervas, I. & Christodoulou, G. (2006). Eletroconvulsoterapia: Critérios e recomendações da Associação Mundial de Psiquiatria. *Review Psiquiatrica Clinicale, 33* (5) 262–267.

[27.] Consoli, A., Benmiloud, M., Wachtel, L., Dhossche, D., Cohen, D. & Bonnot, O. (2010). Electroconvulsive therapy in adolescents with the catatonia syndrome: Efficacy and ethics. *Journal of Electroconvulsive Therapy, 26* (4) 259–265.

[28.] Daly, J. J., Prudic, J., Devanand, D. P., Nobler, M. S., Lisanby, S. H., Peyser, S., Roose, S. P. & Sackheim, H. A. (2001). ECT in bipolar and unipolar depression: Differences in speed of response. *Bipolar Disorder 3* (2) 95–104.

[29.] Kutcher, S. & Robertson, H. A. (1995). Electroconvulsive therapy in treatment resistant bipolar youth. *Journal of Child and Adolescent Psychopharmacology, 5,* 167–175. The authors suggest that electroshock might be an effective and cost-effective treatment in adolescents with bipolar disorder, in acute mania or a depressive state. In 2014 Soreff and colleagues suggested the 'usefulness' of electroshock with patients marked as 'bi-polar'. In 1988 Soreff had been banned from practising medicine in Maine due to sexual relationships with three female patients. He now works in Boston, MA (Soreff., S, McInnes, L & Ahmed, I. (2014). *Bipolar Affective Disorder.* Available at emedicine. medscape.com/article/286342-overview (retrieved 5 August 2014).

30. van Waarde, J. A., Stolker, J. J. & van der Mast, R. C. (2001). ECT in mental retardation: A review. *Journal of Electroconvulsive Therapy, 17* (4) 236–243. The article reviews the literature on the use of electroshock in mental retardation, mostly with those inscribed with 'psychotic depression'. Relapse occurred in half the recipients. See also; Thuppal, M. & Fink, M. (1999). Electroconvulsive therapy and mental retardation. *Journal of Electroconvulsive Therapy 15*, 140–149.

31. Wachtel, L. E., Dhossche, D. M. & Kellner, C. H. (2011). When is electroconvulsive therapy appropriate for children and adolescents? *Medical Hypotheses, 76 (3)* 395– 399; Wachtel, L., Griffin, M. & Reti, I. (2010). Electroconvulsive therapy in a man with autism experiencing severe depression, catatonia, and self-injury. *Journal of Electroconvulsive Therapy, 26 (1)* 70–73.

32. Baeza, I., Flamarique, I., Garrido, J. M., Horga, G., Pons, A., Bernardo, M., Morer, A., Lázaro, M. L., & Castro-Fornieles, J. (2010). Clinical experience using electroconvulsive   therapy   in   adolescents   with

schizophrenia spectrum disorders. *Journal of Child and Adolescent Psychopharmacology, 20 (3)* 205–209.

33. Strober, M., Rao, U., DeAntonio, M., Liston, E., Amaya-Jackson, M., State, L. & Latz, S. (1998). Effects of electroconvulsive therapy in adolescents with severe endogenous depression resistant to pharmacotherapy. *Biological Psychiatry, 43,* 335–338.

34. Walter, G., Koster, K. & Rey, J. M. (1999). Electroconvulsive therapy in adolescents: Experience, knowledge, and attitude of recipients. *Journal of the American Academy of Child and Adolescent Psychiatry, 38,* 594–599.

35. Hale. E. (2009). Child shock therapy. Available at http://intcamp.wordpress.com/ectkids/ (retrieved 8 September 2014).

36. Lima et al, 2013, p. 17. See note 24

37. Jones, Y. & Baldwin, S. (1992). ECT: Shock, lies and psychiatry. *Changes: An international journal of psychology and psychotherapy, 10 (2)* 126–135, p. 134.

38. Collins, J., Halder, N. & Chaudhry, N. (2012). Use of ECT in patients with an intellectual disability: Review. *The Psychiatrist 36,* 55–60.

39. *Ibid.*

40. Aziz, M., Maixner, D. F., DeQuardo, J., Aldridge, A. & Tandon, R. (2001). ECT and mental retardation: A review and case reports. *Journal of Electroconvulsive Therapy, 17,* 149–152.

41. van Waarde J. A., Stolker, J. J. & van der Mast, R. C. (2001). ECT in mental retardation: A review. *Journal of Electroconvulsive Therapy, 17,* 236–243.

42. Herman, R. C., Dorwart, R. A., Hoover, C. W. &

Brody, J. (1995). Variation in ECT use in the United States. *American Journal of Psychiatry, 152*, 869–875; Winslade, W., Liston, E., and Ross, J. (1984). Medical, judicial, and statutory regulations of ECT. *American Journal of Psychiatry, 141,* 1349–1355. This study compared the standards for electroshock recommended by an APA taskforce report and those embodied in federal court orders and state statutes and regulations. The authors conclude that in spite of 'safeguards' promulgated by the psychiatric community, overregulation by legislatures and courts is commonplace. Legal standards can result in 'denials of service' while failing to resolve legal issues involving competence and consent. See also; ECT Statistics (2010). ECT use is not the same everywhere. Available; https:// ectstatistics.wordpress.com/2010/08/19/ect-use-is-not-the-same-everywhere/ (retrieved 18th March 2015).

43. Cassels, C. (2013). ECT in kids: Safe, effective, robust and... underutilized. Available; http://www.medscape.com/viewarticle/806923#3 (retrieved 5 August 2014).

44. APA (2013). The American Psychiatric Association's 2013 Annual Meeting. Abstract NR7-34. Presented 20th May 2013. Available; http://www.medscape.com/viewarticle/806923#3 (retrieved 5 August 2014).

45. *Ibid.*

46. *Ibid.*

47. Coffey, E. C. (1994). The role of structural brain imaging in ECT. *Psychopharmacology Bulletin, 3*, 477–483.

48. Ghaziuddin, N., King, C. A., Naylor, M. W., et al. (1996). Electroconvulsive treatment in adolescents with pharmacotherapy-refractory depression. *Journal of Child and Adolescent Psychopharmacology, 6* (4) 259–271.

49. Szasz, T. (1994) *Cruel Compassion: Psychiatric control of society's unwanted.* New York: John Wiley & Sons

50. *Ibid.*

51. Piper, R. (2018). Fear and loathing in the education system. In. C. Newnes and L. Golding (eds.) *Teaching Critical Psychology: International perspectives.* London: Routledge pp. 82-99

52. ABC News (2014). Electroshock therapy on under-14s banned in WA after law passes Parliament. Available at http://www.abc.net.au/news/2014-10-17/mental-health-billpasses-wa-parliament/5822874 (retrieved 14th March 2015).

53. Aziz et al (2001). See note 40.

54. Spece, R., Shimm, D., and Buchanan, A. (1996). *Conflicts in Clinical and Research Settings.* Oxford: Oxford University Press

55. Baldwin, S. (2001) When 'No' means 'Yes': informed consent themes with children and teenagers. In. C. Newnes, G. Holmes, and C. Dunn (eds.) *This is Madness Too: Critical perspectives on mental health services.* Ross-on-Wye: PCCS Books

56. *Ibid.* p.111

57. Newnes, C. (2016). *Inscription, Diagnosis and Deception in the Mental Health Industry: How Psy governs us all.* Basingstoke: Palgrave Macmillan

[58] Scull, A. (1990). Desperate remedies: A Gothic tale of madness and modern medicine. In. R.M. Murray and T.H. Turner (eds.) *Lectures on the History of Psychiatry: The Squibb Series.* London: Gaskell/Royal College of Psychiatrists pp.144-169 p.155. In 1913 Ferenczi published the case of Arpád, threatened aged five by his father with castration if he ever masturbated. Ferenczi, S. (1913/1916). Ein kleiner Hahnemann translated as A little chanticleer. *Contributions to Psycho-Analysis,* London: Maresfield Library p240.

Zealotry and Zelda Fitzgerald

1. https://ectstatistics.wordpress.com/about/

2. Fennell, P. (1996). *Treatment Without Consent: Law, Psychiatry and the Treatment of Mentally Disordered People Since 1845.* London: Routledge.

3. Valenstein, E. (1986). *Great and Desperate Cures: The Rise and Decline of Psychosurgery and Other Radical Treatments for Mental Illness.* New York: Basic Books.

4. *Ibid.* p.231.

5. See, for example, Lehmann, P. (2010). Medicalization and irresponsibility. *Journal of Critical Psychology, Counselling and Psychotherapy, 10* (4), 209–218.

6. Shorter, E. (2013). Electroconvulsive therapy in children. In. *How Everyone Became Depressed,* http://www.psychologytoday.com/blog/how-everyone -became-depressed/201312/electroconvulsive-therapy-in-children.1December 2013. Retrieved 5th August 2014.

7. https://www.magstim.com/clinical-

solution/0/rapid2-therapy-system

8.Davis, N. (2015). A new milestone in non-pharmaceutical treatments for depression https://www.theguardian.com/science/head-quarters/2015/may/18/non-pharmaceutical-treatments-for-depression-magstim-tms Retrieved. 5 February, 2018.

9.Herwig, M. (1700). *The Art of Curing Sympathetically or Magnetically, Proved to be the Most True by its Theory and Practice*. London: n.p.

10.Carpenter, L.L., Janicak, P.G., Aaronson, S.T., Boyadjis, T., Brock, D.G., Cook, I.A., Dunner, D.L., Lanocha, K., Solvason, H.B., and Demitrack, M.A. (2012). Transcranial magnetic stimulation (TMS) for major depression: a multisite, naturalistic, observational study of acute treatment outcomes in clinical practice. *Depression and Anxiety. 29(7):*587-96. doi: 10.1002/da.21969. Epub 2012 Jun 11. https://www.ncbi.nlm.nih.gov/pubmed/22689344 Retrieved. 26th December, 2017

11. Stein, D. B. (2012). *The Psychology Industry under a Microscope!* Plymouth, UK: University Press of America Inc., p. 1.

12. Carpenter et al. op. cit. p.96.

13.Fitzgerald, Z. (1932/1971) *Save Me the Waltz*. Harmondsworth: Penguin. p.44.

Name index

Bulwer-Lytton, R. (1802-1882) 134

Burstow, B. 246, 336

Burt, C. (1883-1971) 43

Busfield, J. 311

Cattell, R. B. 43-4

Catullus (c.84-54 BCE) 150

Celsus, (c.25BCE – 50 CE) 12

Cerletti, U. (1877–1963) 27, 56-9,62-3, 78, 144, 167, 296

Chasabinski, Ted. 224

Chamberlain, J. 159

Chekhov, A. (1860–1904) 152, 318

Claye Shaw, T. (1841-1927) 77

Cobain, Kurt (1967–1994) 66

Conolly, John (1794-1886) 115

Cooper, D. 153, 250, 337

Cotton, H. (1876-1933) 108, 214-6, 254, 277

Cowes-Prichard, J. (1786-1848) 125

Cromby, J. 217-8, 332

Curie, M. (1867-1934) 253

Dahmer, J. 174

Darwin, C. (1809-1882) 39, 68

Dickens, C. (1812-1870) 150, 227-8

Dörner, A. 121

Duchenne, G-B-A, (1806-1875) 7, 75

Eastwood, Clint. 144

Ellis, Havelock. (1859-1939) 180-1, 190, 337

Engels, F. (1820–1895) 151

Erb, W. H. (1840-1921) 75

Esquirol, J–E, D. (1772–1840) 85, 250

Eysenck, H. (1916–1997) 207

Faith, K. 144, 245

Subject index

Electricity and Medicine 6

electrocution 7, 20, 47, 55-60, 69, 81-2, 133, 139, 219-221, 233, 251, 256-7, 281

electroshock statistics
    California 106, 246
    England 50-1, 128, 247
    Texas 107, 121, 246
    United Kingdom 256
    World 88, 256

elephant 55-6

epilepsy 6, 56-7, 74, 77, 249-50, 253

Equanil 223

eugenics 43, 242

European Network of Users and Survivors of Psychiatry; ENUSP 160

exhaustion 20, 75, 82, 244

experimentation 11, 47-8, 69, 127, 189, 253

exploitation 11, 47, 151
    of minors 274

Facebook 15, 140, 146-7, 158
    and illusion 225

fear 30, 42, 70, 217, 255

Federal Bureau of Investigation; FBI 79

Federal Drug Agency; FDA 125

fever therapy 164

First People 201, 242

focal infection 108, 214, 254

gas chamber 41

gaze (le Regard) 37, 68, 71, 117, 124, 245

genocide 44, 93, 293

gin 155

The Real Press

By the same author...

If you enjoyed this book, take a look at the other books we have on our list at www.therealpress.co.uk

Including the new Armada novel with a difference, *Tearagh't*, by the maverick psychologist Craig Newnes. Also his latest novel, a psychological love story tragedy, set in Paris, partly today and partly in an authentic Hundred Years' War.

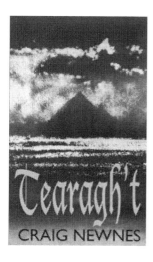
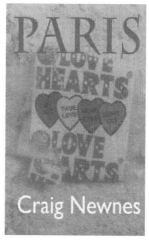

25692301R00222

Printed in Great Britain
by Amazon